TREAT YOUR OWN HIP™

ROBIN MCKENZIE

CNZM,OBE, FCSP (Hon), FNZSP (Hon),
DipMDT, Dip MT

with Grant Watson

NZSP, ADP (OMT), Dip MT, Dip MDT

and Robert Lindsay

NZSP, ADP (OMT),Dip MT

McKENZIE GLOBAL LTD.

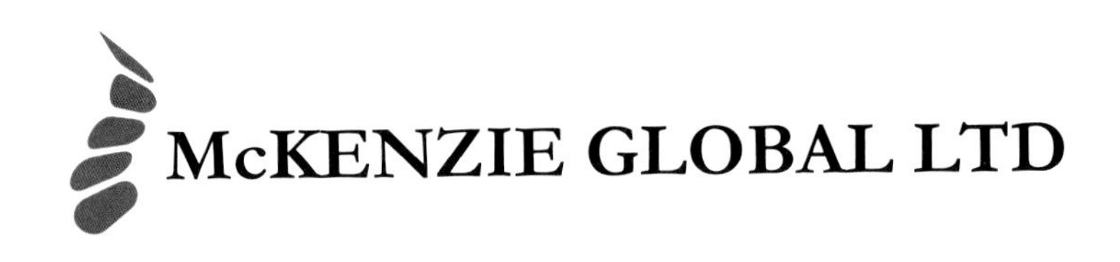

Treat Your Own Hip

First Edition published in 2019
1st U.S. edition, A5 portrait, 2020

McKenzie Global Ltd

info@mckenziemethod.com
www.mckenziemethod.com
Telephone: +64 4 299 7020

ISBN: 978-1-942798-20-0

Designed by Gregory Studio, New Zealand – gregorystudio.com
Typeset by Tina Delceg
Copy edited by Judith Watson
Photography by Daniel Allen

Stock photography by www.shutterstock.com and www.istockphoto.com
Exclusively distributed by OPTP in the U.S. and Canada - OPTP.com
Printed in the USA

About the authors and this book

Robin McKenzie

The late Robin McKenzie was born in Auckland, New Zealand, in 1931. He graduated from the New Zealand School of Physiotherapy in 1952 and thereafter specialised in the treatment of spinal disorders.

During the course of the 1960s and 70s McKenzie developed his own specific examination and treatment methods, later known as The McKenzie Method®, for a range of musculoskeletal complaints. Viewed as radical at its inception, the McKenzie Method® of Mechanical Diagnosis and Therapy®, also known as MDT™, has since received international recognition and acclaim and is now taught and practised by medical professionals worldwide. Indeed, in 2004, the Orthopaedic Section of the American Physical Therapists Association voted Robin McKenzie: "the most influential physical therapist or physician, of all time".

Central to the McKenzie Method® is the contention that 'self-management and self- treatment' of most musculoskeletal complaints is more effective, in the long-term, than any other treatment method. In accordance with that contention, during the 1980s, Robin McKenzie began writing a series of self-help books, the Treat Your Own Series, which includes *Treat Your Own Back*, *Treat Your Own Neck*, *Treat Your Own Shoulder* and *Treat Your Own Knee*.

In the course of these books McKenzie sought to distil the essence of his 'method', as taught to medical professionals globally, in an easy-to-follow format, so that it would be accessible directly to the sufferer, without recourse to a clinician. Each book contains an easy-to-understand treatment plan to alleviate pain and maintain joint health, through the inexpensive, non-invasive and clinically proven McKenzie Method®. Essentially, the reader is guided through a detailed assessment of their pain and then provided with a series of simple exercises to correct and restore their mobility.

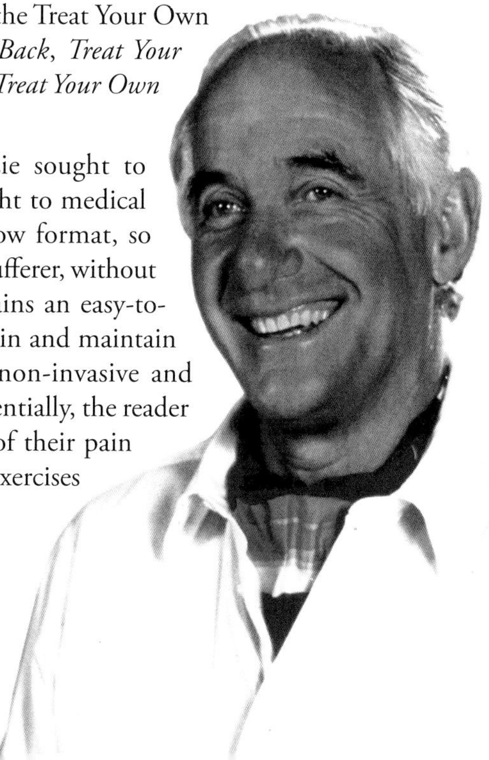

The McKenzie Method® has attracted intense interest from researchers all over the world. It is acknowledged that the methods described have helped millions of people worldwide take control of their own pain and postural management, avoid surgery, minimise investigations, and prevent a long-term costly dependency upon clinicians. Since initial publication the books have been translated into some 18 languages and are consistently global best sellers.

In the process of developing his 'method' for self-treatment, McKenzie also came to realise that correct spinal supports were "vital for many of my patients, if they were to remain pain free". Initially McKenzie designed a lumbar roll that his wife, Joy, "made on our kitchen table", but with numerous patients confirming their efficacy, he then set about designing and developing a specialised range of portable spinal supports, which would cater to different needs. Of detailed and specific design, made of durable, high-quality, materials, The Original McKenzie® range of rolls complement the exercises in the books, assist in postural management and alleviate pain. They are the only lumbar supports approved for use with the McKenzie Method®. For further information on the books and rolls and how to acquire them, please refer to the website: OPTP.com.

As stated above, Robin McKenzie's ground-breaking work has received accolades from scientific and medical communities around the world. During his lifetime he was awarded numerous honorary memberships and fellowships of international medical associations: "in recognition of distinguished and meritorious service to the art and science of physical therapy, and to the welfare of mankind" (The American Physical Therapy Association). His outstanding contribution was also recognised by Her Majesty Queen Elizabeth II, in the award of an OBE (Officer of the Most Excellent Order of the British Empire) in 1990 followed by a CNZM (Companion of the New Zealand Order of Merit) in 2000.

These extraordinary and wonderful tributes essentially reflect Robin McKenzie's selfless determination to put the patient first and thereby to empower self care.

Grant Watson

Grant Watson is a Physiotherapist in Golden Bay, New Zealand. He has been a Senior and International Instructor, and Assistant Director of Education, for the McKenzie Institute International and has represented the Institute extensively in many corners of the world since 1995. He has been actively involved with education within physiotherapy since 1985, and for many years was an Accredited Physiotherapist to the New Zealand Academy of Sport. He is co-author with Robin McKenzie of *Treat Your Own Shoulder* (2009), *Treat Your Own Knee* (2012), and co-author of *Treat Your Own Strains, Sprains and Bruises* (1994). In 2012 he was awarded the 'Bronze Lady' Extension Award in recognition of his outstanding contribution to education in the field of Mechanical Diagnosis and Therapy.

Robert Lindsay

Robert Lindsay is a Physiotherapist in Private Practice in Coromandel Peninsula, New Zealand with postgraduate qualifications in orthopedic and manipulative physiotherapy. He firmly believes in the role of education and self treatment within the scope of physiotherapy, as people generally are able to successfully treat and prevent or limit recurrence of many of the soft tissue disorders that occur in daily life. He is co-author with Robin McKenzie of *Treat Your Own Shoulder* (2009), *Treat Your Own Knee* (2012), and co-author of *Treat Your Own Strains, Sprains and Bruises* (1994).

Acknowledgements

The authors would like to thank:

Alistair McKenzie and the McKenzie family for their support in continuing to develop the legacy of Robin McKenzie. Richard Rosedale and Rob Hughes for contributing their extensive expertise in the McKenzie Method to the information in this book, and to the MII Education Council for assistance with early drafts of the manuscript. We would also like to thank Jude Watson for her editing, Daniel Allen for his photography, and to acknowledge the creative expertise of our designer, Tina Delceg who made the final stages of this book preparation a pleasure. Robbie Burton of Potton & Burton Publishing has been a huge support in the background, and recommended the aforementioned experts in their respective fields. Finally, we would like to thank the thousands of patients who unknowingly provided most of the solutions for hip pain that are described in this book.

Books by Robin McKenzie

Mobilisation of the Spinal Column
Kaltenborn, F.M. Technical translation by McKenzie,R.
Wellington, N.Z. : New Zealand University Press,
Price Milburn, 1970.

Treat Your Own Back™ (now in its 9th edition)
McKenzie, R. Waikanae, N.Z.: McKenzie Global Ltd,
First published 1980.

Lumbar Spine: Mechanical Diagnosis and Therapy
McKenzie, R. Waikanae, N.Z.:
Spinal Publications NZ Ltd, 1981.

Treat Your Own Neck™ (now in its 5th edition)
McKenzie, R. Waikanae, N.Z.: McKenzie Global Ltd,
First published 1983.

Cervical and Thoracic Spine: Mechanical Diagnosis and Therapy
McKenzie, R. Waikanae, N.Z.:
Spinal Publications NZ Ltd, 1990.

Extremities: Mechanical Diagnosis and Therapy
McKenzie, R and May, S. Waikanae, N.Z.:
Spinal Publications NZ Ltd, 2000.

7 Steps to a Pain Free Life
McKenzie, R and Kubey, C. New York: Plume, 2001.

The Lumbar Spine: Mechanical Diagnosis and Therapy, 2nd ed.
McKenzie, R and May, S. Waikanae, N.Z.:
Spinal Publications NZ Ltd, 2003.

The Cervical and Thoracic Spine: Mechanical Diagnosis and Therapy, 2nd ed.
McKenzie, R and May, S. Raumati Beach, N.Z.:
Spinal Publications NZ Ltd, 2006.

Against the Tide: Back pain treatment – the breakthrough: An Autobiography
McKenzie, R with Bybee, R. Wellington, N.Z.:
Dunmore Publishing, 2009.

Treat Your Own Shoulder™
McKenzie, R with Watson, G and Lindsay, R.
Raumati Beach, N.Z.: McKenzie Global Ltd,
First published 2009.

Treat Your Own Knee™
McKenzie, R with Watson, G and Lindsay, R.
Raumati Beach, N.Z.: McKenzie Global Ltd,
First published 2012.

Treat Your Own Hip™
McKenzie, R., Watson, G., Lindsay, R.
Waikanae, N.Z.: McKenzie Global Ltd, 2019.
First published 2019.

Contents

About the authors and this book 3

Acknowledgements 6

Books by Robin McKenzie 7

Chapter 1: Introduction 12

Hip Problems 12

Osteoarthritis, degeneration or normal wear and tear? 12

Is the pain inevitable? 13

MRIs – do they tell the full story ? 13

Myths 14

Hip pain 14

Is the information in this book suitable for me? 18

Diagnosing your problem 19

Who can perform self-treatment? 26

Chapter 2: Understanding the hip region 30

The hip 30

Functions of the hip region 30

Mechanical pain 30

Mechanical hip pain 35

Tissue damage 35

Chapter 3: Common causes of hip pain 38

1. Inactivity–low fitness levels 39

2. Postural stresses 42

Postural neglect 43

Prolonged sitting postures 43

Prolonged standing postures 44

Lying and sleeping 45

3. Being overweight..46
Lateral hip pain 47
Ongoing pain and reduced function following hip surgery...............48
Chapter 4: Understanding the McKenzie Method® 50
The aim of the exercises 50
Effect on pain intensity and location 50
Pain intensity 51
Starting the exercise programme..52
Chapter 5: The exercise programme 54
Overview..54
If you are in significant pain 54
When acute or severe pain has subsided..55
To start this process of recovery 55
Exercise 1: Hip extension in kneeling...55
Review your progress...58
Exercise 2: Hip flexion in sitting 58
Exercise 3: Hip abduction and lateral rotation in sitting...................61
Alternative: sitting position in a chair 61
Review your progress...63
No response or benefit..63
Lateral hip pain 64
Exercise 4: Hip strengthening – hip abduction in standing...............64
Exercise 5: Hip strengthening in standing – two-legged half squat.....65
Review your progress...67
When you have no pain or stiffness 68
Recurrence 71
Ongoing hip pain following hip surgery 71

Chapter 6: Acute management and prevention of recurrence 74
Acute management.......74
Prevention of recurrence.......76
1. Interrupt prolonged sitting and standing postures regularly.......77
2. Increase the amount you walk 78
3. Increase your general fitness.......79
4. Improve your balance.......80
5. Lose weight.......82
References.......86
The McKenzie Institute International.......87
Licensed Distributors.......88

Under certain circumstances throughout this book, where difficulties may arise in your progress, you are referred to the website: www.mckenzieinstitute.org. Here you will find details on how to find a clinician that has been Credentialed or Diplomaed by the McKenzie Institute International. These are the only approved clinicians qualified to deliver the McKenzie Method® of Mechanical Diagnosis and Therapy.

Chapter 1: Introduction

Hip problems

Compared to ankle and knee injuries, hip pain is less common when we are young and generally more active. At any age the hip may be injured in a heavy fall or in a sporting activity; however it is in our middle to later years that hip pain usually starts to appear and affect our lives.

Hip pain affects our ability to do daily tasks like getting up from sitting, getting in and out of the car, or putting on socks or shoes. Going up and down steps or stairs becomes difficult, and we can develop a limp that causes pain to occur in other areas as the body tries to compensate. Many of us assume immediately it is the development of osteoarthritis of the hip, and that we are potentially looking at a hip replacement sooner rather than later.

The incidence of people reporting hip pain is around 10 per cent of the 40–50-year-old age group, increasing to around 25 per cent of over 65 year olds. Hip problems are often referred to in different ways, including osteoarthritis (OA), bursitis, trochanteric bursitis, labral tear, impingement syndrome, or tendinitis or groin strain.

Osteoarthritis, degeneration or normal aging changes?

While it is possible to injure our hips by twisting or falling, or through overuse such as a sudden increase in activity, most recurrent hip pain in adults appears to occur for no apparent reason, and is commonly diagnosed by health professionals as 'osteoarthritis'.

The American Academy of Orthopaedic Surgeons and other associated groups report that more than 27 million people have osteoarthritis of the hip in the USA, with numbers increasing steadily. The incidence of total hip joint replacement surgery also continues to increase around the world. However, this diagnosis is often based almost solely on an X-ray looking for aging changes in the joints, which are evident in up to 70 per cent of the population over 50 years old.

But, as in other areas of the body, evidence of aging changes on an X-ray is not a very accurate guide as to whether pain or disability will be present. The most commonly used term to describe these aging changes is 'degeneration', when in fact it is usually no more than normal wear and tear. They are part of a normal aging process and may not be the cause of pain. For example, we may complain of pain in one hip joint, yet find the same aging changes if we X-ray both hips for a comparison. The assumption that this 'degeneration' is causing the hip pain becomes questionable when so many cases start improving by applying the self-treatment methods described in this book.

Is the pain inevitable?

Similarly, we tend to believe the pain from osteoarthritis will be slowly progressive, and that becoming worse is inevitable. However, several studies show that, in a number of people, symptoms get no worse or they actually improve over time, even as the X-ray changes show deterioration over the same period. This book will give you the information to do everything you can to make that improvement.

The Cochrane Database of Systematic Reviews concludes that scientific evidence demonstrates land-based therapeutic exercise programmes can decrease pain and increase physical function amongst people with symptomatic hip osteoarthritis.

MRIs – do they tell the full story?

Hip osteoarthritis is most commonly diagnosed by an X-ray. Magnetic Resonance Imaging (MRI) scans are another imaging tool used to diagnose sources of hip pain because of their ability to reveal the appearance of apparent damage to the structures in and around the hip. However, MRI scans do not always give us an exact picture of the site or severity of the injury, or give clear guidance for treatment strategies. Many studies show experts disagree on the interpretation of MRIs, and other studies show surgeons often find MRI findings inaccurate when they perform the surgery. Also, there is evidence to show that in many cases the findings are not clinically relevant. A 2011 study on young elite hockey players with no hip symptoms found 77 per cent had MRI findings indicating hip or groin tissue damage.

While some cases of hip pain do require surgery, all of the **guidelines on hip pain** around the world recommend avoiding surgery if possible by first exploring self-management options such as education and exercises.

Myths

There are many myths associated with aging changes in the hip.

These relate either to the **cause**:

- "I must have over-used my hip due to years of running or hiking for recreation."
- "My occupation requires me to be active and my hips are getting worn out."

or they relate to **management**:

- "Now I have osteoarthritis I must rest the hip by doing less."
- "Due to my age and pain, I should consider a hip replacement sooner rather than later."

In fact none of the above are correct. The truth is, most of us are not consistently active enough in our adult lives to maintain the flexibility and strength required for full hip function. It is not the more active people who consistently report hip pain but those who have a more sedentary lifestyle or who have become overweight. The expression "If you don't use it, you lose it" clearly relates to the health of all the joints of the body and the surrounding muscles.

The single most effective management for hip pain of mechanical origin in most people is actually increasing the amount of appropriate exercise they give to their hips, and gradually increasing overall activity and fitness.

Hip pain

Hip pain can be felt in a variety of ways. There may be some pain or stiffness in both hips, although usually one hip is more troublesome than the other. There can be days or times in the day when there is no pain felt. Symptoms of pain or stiffness may appear for no apparent reason, and just as mysteriously disappear or change location. Sometimes the symptoms may only occur with specific movements of the hip; at other times the pain and stiffness appear when standing or lying on the painful hip for prolonged periods. Therefore, it is also common for hip pain to regularly disturb your sleep. This pain and stiffness may be felt to some degree at all times throughout the day. People who have pain all of the time are frequently forced to take medication and sometimes have to stop work or give up certain hobbies such as hiking or golf. The pain simply makes their lives miserable, and they have to reduce their activities in order to keep the discomfort at a manageable level. However, the consequence of this is they start to lose fitness and gain weight, further impacting on their hip problem.

If you have problems of this nature, you may have already discovered that the symptoms can last for months or even years. You may have found that some treatments decrease or stop your pain temporarily, but the pain returns later when you try to return to your normal activities. You may be reading this book because you have persistent hip pain that limits some of your activities and has not improved, despite the fact you may have received many types of treatments.

Common treatments for hip pain are medication, injections, surgery, acupuncture, or electrical modalities such as ultrasound, TENS and interferential therapy. However, whilst some of these treatments may appear to have short-term benefits, there is no strong evidence that they provide effective long-term relief from pain and loss of function. Similarly, following an extensive review of many studies, the American Academy of Orthopaedic Surgeons does not support the widely advertised nutritional supplements such as glucosamine or chondroitin sulphate. Although these do no harm, they do not get to the real cause of pain and are no better than placebo treatment in some studies.

The 2008 Osteoarthritis Research Society International recommendations for hip and knee pain clearly state: "The initial focus should be on self-help and patient-driven treatments rather than on passive therapies delivered by health professionals".

You may also have been given exercises to perform, and perhaps you have found these to be of some benefit. However, many people do not realise that stretching and strengthening your muscles alone does not

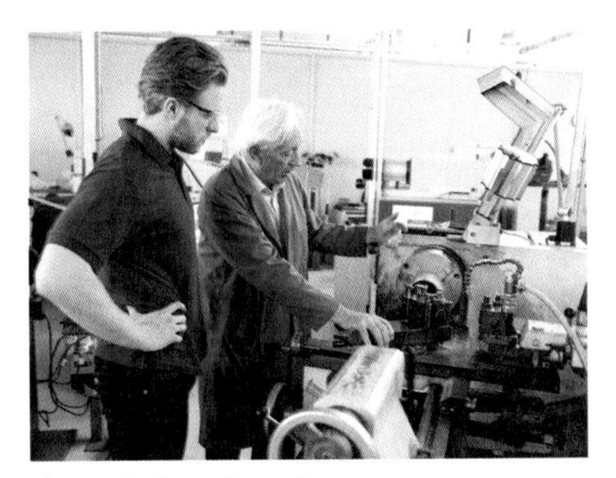

Photo 1 Prolonged standing

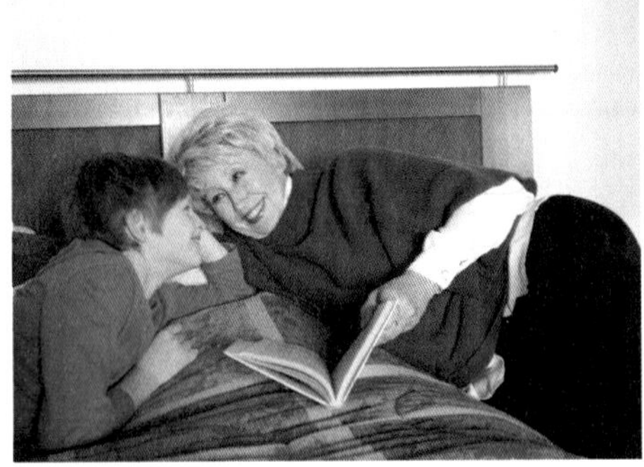

Photo 2 Lying on painful side

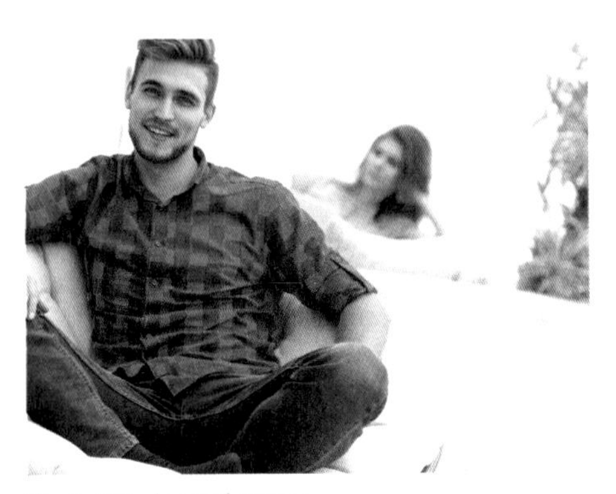

Photo 3 Prolonged sitting

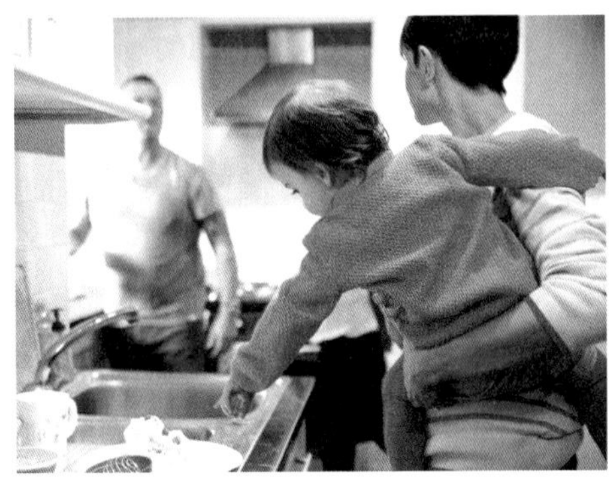

Photo 4 Carrying weight unevenly

automatically give you relief from hip pain. 'Doing your exercises' is only part of the solution; what we seldom consider are the other aggravating factors that contribute to your hip pain.

It is important to understand how prolonged static positions or postures you adopt during activities, or within your occupation, such as prolonged standing as a factory worker (*Photo 1*), or lying on the painful side (*Photo 2*) can significantly contribute to your hip problem. Prolonged sitting with your hips bent (*Photo 3*), or carrying a weight on one side (*Photo 4*) can also aggravate the pain if these positions are not regularly interrupted.

Whatever the situation, you may have realised many of the treatments dispensed by doctors and physical therapists are prescribed for your present symptoms and not directed at preventing future problems. Time and again you may have to seek assistance to get relief from your hip pain. How satisfying would it be to apply treatment to yourself whenever pain arose? Better still, to apply a system of treatment to yourself that would prevent or reduce the onset of pain? The most important thing for most people is to remain active, understand and apply the self-management strategies as described in this book and, where indicated, lose some body weight.

Since the 1970s, methods have been discovered for how to manage our own spinal and extremity problems. The self-treatment methods we describe here evolved after Robin McKenzie's experiences with more than 20,000 patients during 40 years of practice. The methods have been used for neck and low back pain by doctors and physical therapists in many parts of the world for decades. Millions of people have found relief by putting into practice what they read in the first two books in this series: *Treat Your Own Back*, first published in 1980, and *Treat Your Own Neck* (1983). Both books have been translated into many languages, and are still selling strongly. This same McKenzie approach has been used for 'mechanical' pain in other regions of the body, such as the shoulder, knee and hip. Satisfactory results with many patients led to the publication of *Treat Your Own Shoulder* in 2009 and *Treat Your Own Knee* in 2012.

More than 40 years ago, Robin McKenzie stated that health-care professionals have a duty to provide accurate information to patients about self-managing their own condition, and that patients have the right to receive this information. Groups such as the Osteoarthritis Research Society International and the National Institute of Health and Clinical Excellence in UK now realise the "importance of good communication between patients and health-care professionals, promoting evidence-based information tailored to each patient's needs".

It has been shown repeatedly that patients require a rational explanation for their problems. They need education about the postures, activities and exercises that allow them to remain free of disabling symptoms. They need advice on how to avoid or manage the detrimental forces encountered in daily living and how to apply beneficial strategies and lifestyle changes. All of these things are found in this book.

One of the key messages of *Treat Your Own Hip* is that the management of your hip is best accomplished by you. If for some reason you have developed a hip problem, then you must learn how to deal with the present symptoms and how to prevent or limit future problems.

Self-treatment will be more effective in the long-term management of your hip pain than any other form of treatment because you can self-treat multiple times a day. It is the least expensive treatment and safer than receiving treatment from other people. **Self-management gives you the tools to get better and to stay better.**

Is the information in this book suitable for me?

The advice given in this book is provided for those people with straightforward, recurring mechanical problems of the hip. You can commence the exercise programme, provided the recommended precautions have been taken as described later in this chapter.

However, you should *not* commence the exercise programme without first consulting your doctor or physical therapist, if you:

- have severe pain in your back, and in the thigh or leg, and experience sensations of weakness, numbness or pins and needles in the thigh, leg or foot
- have suddenly developed severe hip pain following a recent accident and find you are unable to take any weight through your leg or it keeps collapsing for no reason
- are feeling generally unwell in conjunction with your hip pain
- have a previous history of cancer or a tumour
- have had hip surgery in the past six months
- are a child or adolescent who has developed hip, groin, thigh or knee pain, or have developed a limp with or without any specific injury

If you have developed hip pain for the first time, follow the instructions and guidelines over the next several pages.

If you have any doubt about your suitability for this self-management programme, we recommend you consult your doctor or physical therapist before commencing.

It pays to choose your therapist carefully. You should be provided with the information and education you require to manage your own problem. Every patient deserves to have the opportunity to learn how to manage their own hip problem, and every therapist should be obligated to provide that information. This is the essence of the McKenzie Method®.

The only health-care professionals fully qualified to provide the McKenzie Method® are members of the McKenzie Institute International who hold the credentialing certificate or the Diploma in Mechanical Diagnosis & Therapy®. To obtain names of these treatment providers in your area use the McKenzie Institute International website: www.mckenzieinstitute.org.

The information provided in *Treat Your Own Hip* will enable you to determine with reasonable certainty whether your hip is the source of your pain, and if you will benefit from the methods outlined in this book.

Once you have started the exercises, carefully watch your pain pattern. If your pain is getting progressively worse and remains worse the following day, or if it is slowly increasing in severity and becoming intolerable, you should seek advice from your doctor or a McKenzie Institute International clinician to learn alternative exercises or to consider other treatment strategies.

Diagnosing your problem

The role of the low back in hip pain

The hip has a close relationship with the low back or lumbar region of the spine, and commonly the pain and loss of movement we feel in our hip is actually coming from a problem in our low back. Therefore, with all hip problems it is important to attempt to exclude the low back as the source of the pain. Even with the use of X-rays, ultrasound scans and MRI scans, health professionals can have difficulty identifying the specific source of the pain in the hip region due to its close involvement with the spine and pelvis. In fact, the emphasis is often on labelling the patient's condition despite the lack of an exact idea of the site or severity of the injury, with a resulting lack of clear guidance for treatment strategies.

"Is my pain coming from my hip or low back?"

Very commonly, pain that is felt in the hip may be coming from a source in the low back region of the lumbar spine. This is explained in more detail later in this chapter to help you decide whether it is your hip or your back which is the issue. But it is important to note that it is uncommon for it to be BOTH a low back problem and a separate hip problem.

Here are three important questions to consider:

1. Do you have pain in your central low back area, and particularly back pain on the same side as the hip pain?
2. Does coughing or sneezing produce or increase your hip or back pain?
3. Do you have any areas of numbness, pins and needles, or weakness in the knee or foot on the same side as your hip pain?

If you answered YES to any of these questions, it is likely your pain is coming from your low back, and we recommend you read *Treat Your Own Back* in this series before continuing with the programme described in this book.

However, if you answered NO to the questions, read on. You will have another opportunity to decide whether this book is suitable for you later in this chapter.

The two most reliable indicators to determine whether the pain is coming from structures in the low back or the hip are:

1. pain location
2. pain behaviour

Pain location

The sites of pain caused by both hip or low back problems can be similar in some cases. As a general rule, pain originating in the hip will be felt in the outside or front of the hip, or in the groin, and may be associated with stiffness or weakness. This general hip pain may on occasion radiate down towards the thigh or knee (*Figure 1*), but it is uncommon for affected hip structures to cause pain at the back of the hip or to radiate upwards into the low back area (*Figure 2*). However, it is possible for back pain to radiate downwards towards the hip, and even into the knee or foot. (*Figure 3*). Similarly, a hip problem will not give you a sensation of pins and needles or numbness in the leg or foot. These symptoms are much more likely to be referred from the low back.

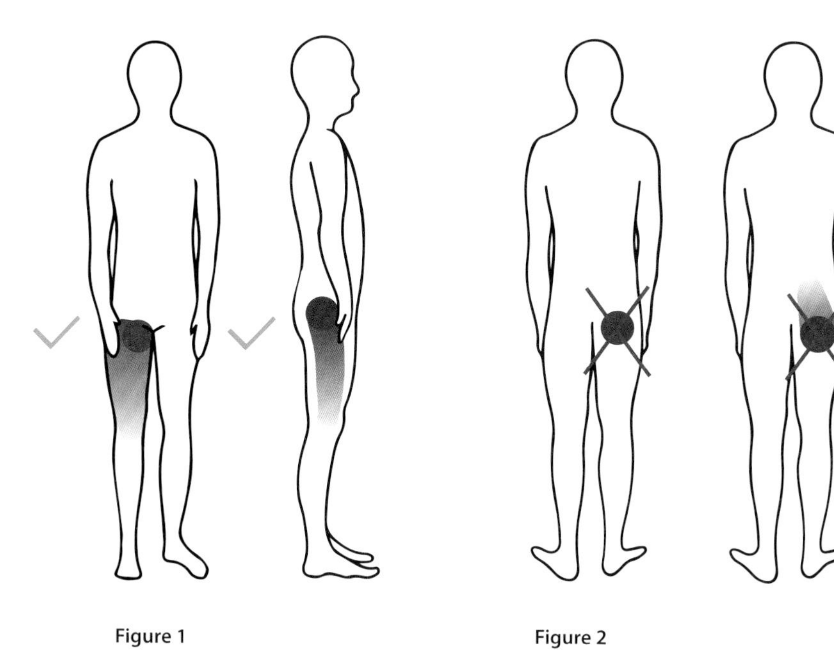
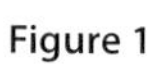

Figure 1

Figure 2

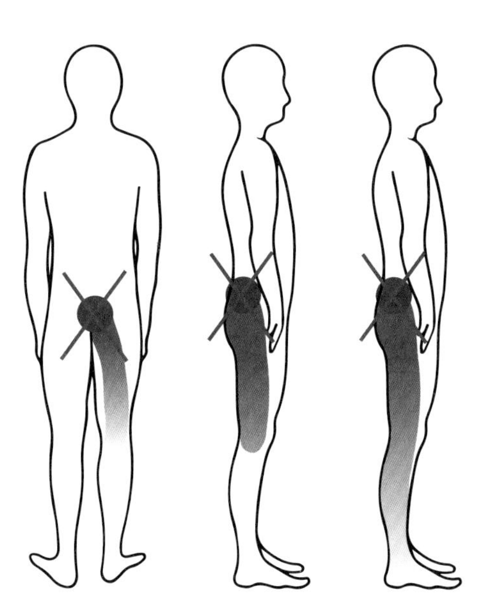

Figure 3

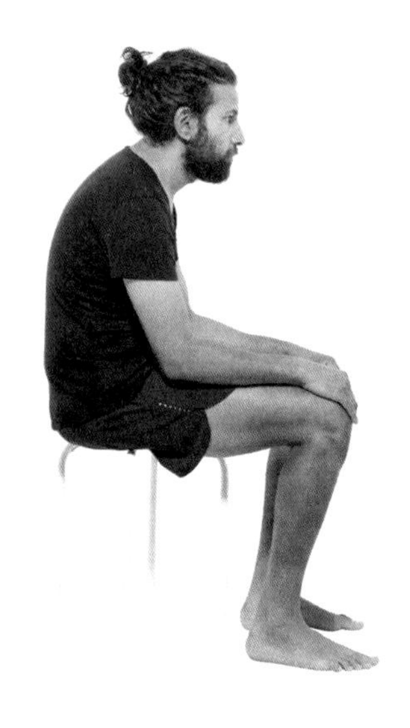

Photo 5 Slouched sitting posture

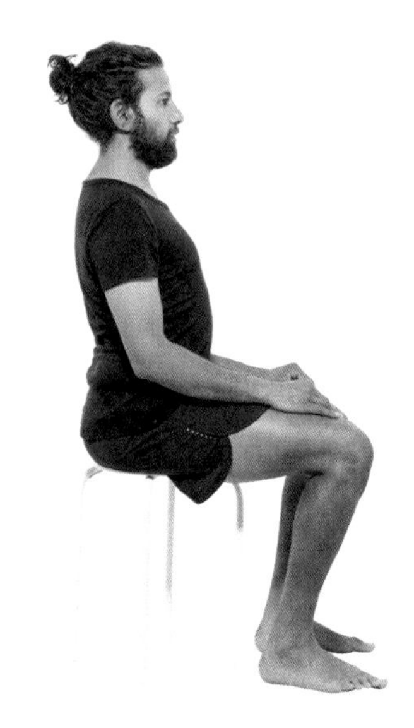

Photo 6 Extreme of sitting position

Pain behaviour

In most cases, pain originating from the structures in and around the hip is produced or aggravated by moving the hip and leg – particularly during walking, or by rotating or moving the hip sideways to get in and out of bed, or drying the feet, for example. Hip pain originating from the low back is frequently altered by low back positions or movements. To determine whether low back movements affect your hip pain, we recommend you perform the following test movements, carefully noting any change in your pain location and intensity:

Sit on a stool of chair height or sideways on a kitchen or dining chair. Allow yourself to slouch completely (*Photo 5*). Relax for up to 30 seconds in the slouched position and monitor the intensity and location of your hip pain. Now move slowly up into an upright position and accentuate the curve in your back (it is called a lordosis) until you are in the extreme of the sitting position (*Photo 6*).

If these low back **postures** have no effect on your hip pain it is probable that the hip is the source of your pain. However, if these low back positions change the intensity of the pain, or the location of your hip pain towards or away from your back, the source of your pain may be the structures in your low back.

To further determine whether back **movements** affect your hip pain, we recommend you perform the following test movements, shown to be a reliable guide to identifying symptoms that arise in the back.

You may or may not have pain at this time around your hip, or in the groin or thigh, but you should have no back pain as previously discussed. If you have pain or aching remember the position and intensity of your symptoms at this point. Monitor your pain as you move and also after the last of the bending movements to see if the location or intensity have changed.

1. Back flexion in standing (bending forward)

   Stand upright with your feet about shoulder-width apart, and allow your arms to hang loosely by your side. Bend forward and run your hands down your legs as far as you can comfortably reach while keeping your legs straight. Maintain this position for 1 or 2 seconds, then return to the upright position. Repeat this exercise up to 10 times slowly and rhythmically, trying to bend a little bit further each time, returning each time to the upright position. (*Photos 7 and 8*)

2. Back extension in standing (arching backwards)

   Stand upright with your feet shoulder-width apart, and your hands in the small of your back with the fingertips pointing backwards so they meet in the centre of your spine. Bend your trunk backwards from the waist as far as you can using your hands as the pivot point. It is important to try and keep your knees straight. Maintain this position for 1 or 2 seconds, then return to the upright position. Repeat this exercise up to 10 times slowly and rhythmically, trying to bend a little bit further back each time, returning each time to the upright position. (*Photos 9 and 10*)

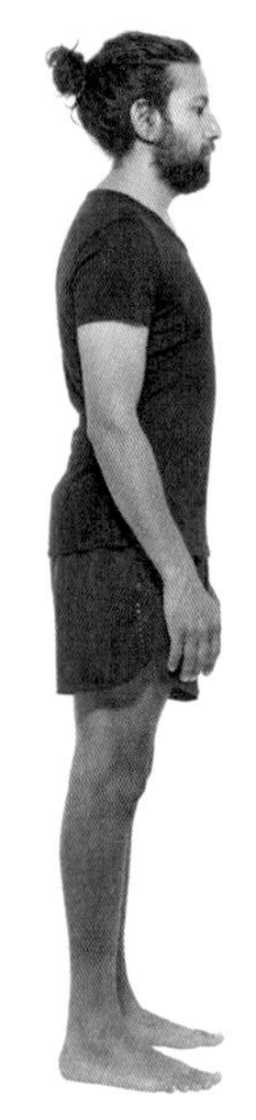

Photo 7 Standing upright

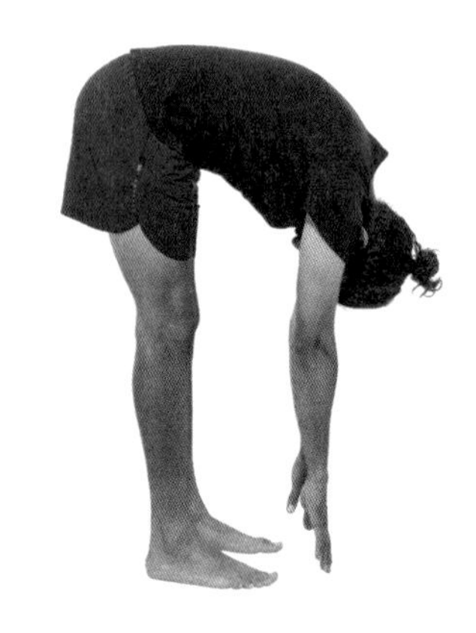

Photo 8 Flexion

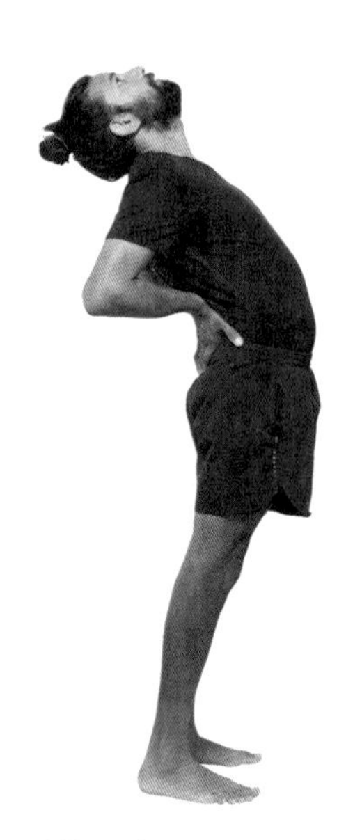

Photo 9 Extension

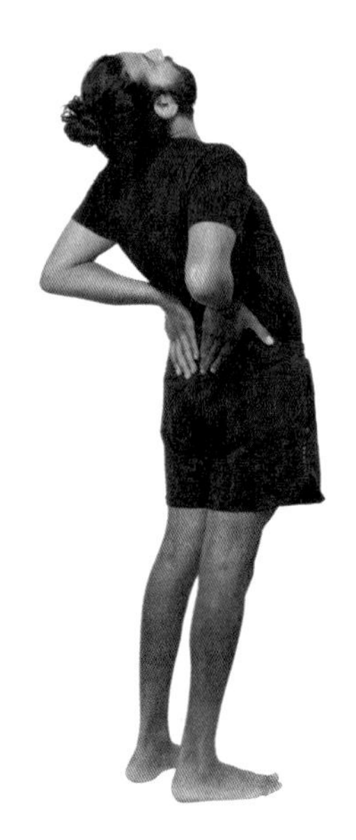

Photo 10 Oblique view

3. Side gliding (glide hips to one side whilst attempting to keep your shoulders level)

   Stand upright with your feet shoulder-width apart, and your hands on your hips. Glide your pelvis away from your painful hip as far as you comfortably can (*Photo 11*). Maintain this position for 1 or 2 seconds, then return to the starting position. Repeat this exercise up to 10 times slowly and rhythmically, trying to side glide a little bit further each time, returning each time to the starting position.

   Then repeat the side gliding movement of your pelvis in the opposite direction. (*Photo 12*)

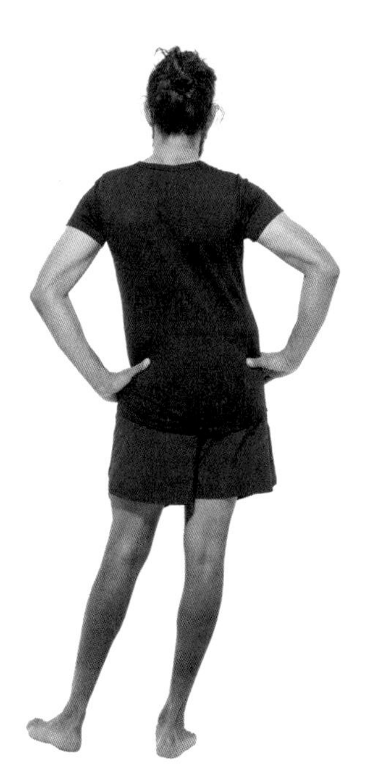

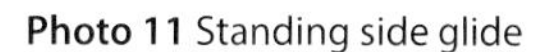

Photo 11 Standing side glide

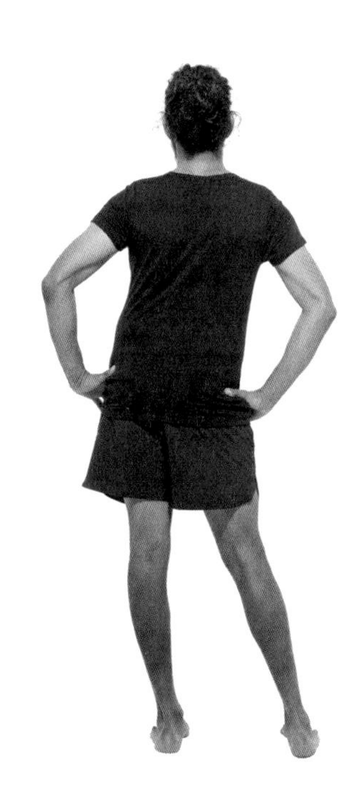

Photo 12 Opposite side glide

These postures or movements primarily load the spine and can be a reliable guide to the source of your pain. If none of these repeated movements of your back has any effect on your hip pain it is probable the hip is the source of your pain. However, if any of these repeated movements of your back appear to either produce back pain or alter the location of your hip pain to or away from your back, the source of the pain is probably the structures in your low back. In this case we recommend that you read *Treat Your Own Back* instead.

Who can perform self-treatment?

Having determined that your hip region is the source of your pain, we recommend you spend a few minutes completing the following checklist. Answering all the questions will determine whether you can treat your hip successfully without further assistance:

	Yes	No
1. Are there periods in the day when you have no pain or aching? Even ten minutes?	☐	☐
2. Do you have pain when you walk up or down stairs or hills?	☐	☐
3. Have you had several episodes of hip pain over the past months or years?	☐	☐
4. Between episodes, is your hip pain-free?	☐	☐
5. When your hip is painful, does it feel as if you are unable to fully move it in all directions compared to your unaffected hip – such as when drying your feet?	☐	☐
6. Between episodes, are you able to fully move your hip more freely in all directions with less pain? Are you generally able to walk without limping?	☐	☐
7. Is the pain localised to the area around the hip joint or groin?	☐	☐
8. Are you generally worse when getting out of a chair and with the first few steps walking after prolonged sitting?	☐	☐
9. Are some days better or worse than others?	☐	☐
10. Do you have pain when lying on the side of the painful hip, but some nights are better or worse than others?	☐	☐

If you answered:

- **'Yes' to all of the above questions** you are an ideal candidate for the self-treatment outlined in this book.
- **'Yes' to five or more questions**, your chances to benefit from self-treatment are good and you should commence the programme.
- **'Yes' to only four or fewer questions** then some form of specialised treatment may be required and you should consult the directory included at the back of the book for a therapist credentialed or diplomaed by the McKenzie Institute International. Or you can use the search feature on the McKenzie Institute International website: www.mckenzieinstitute.org.

This book describes a complete system of management, which must be followed in its entirety to ensure success. Do not turn straight to the exercise description pages; your understanding of Chapters One to Four is essential.

NOTES

Chapter 2: Understanding the hip region

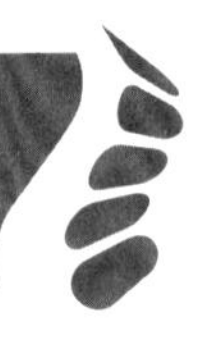

The hip

The hip is a ball-and-socket joint between the pelvis and the thigh bone – the femur. On the outer aspect of the femur close to the hip joint is a bony prominence called the greater trochanter, to which several muscle groups from the pelvis attach.

The joint surface of the pelvis, known as the acetabulum, and the joint surface of the femur are covered with a substance called articular cartilage, which gives a smooth protective coating to the surface of the joint, similar to the surface of a ball bearing. The acetabulum also has a cartilage rim known as a labrum, which provides a greater contact surface for the hip joint (*Figure 4*).

The hip joint itself is surrounded by a sack-like structure, called a capsule, which assists in supporting the hip joint. It also contains the lubricating fluid that circulates through the hip joint to assist with its nutrition (*Figure 5*).

The outer aspect of the hip has several muscle groups from the pelvis that attach in and around the greater trochanter (*Figure 6*). These muscles absorb a significant amount of force during weight-bearing movement, for example when walking, using stairs or running, and sometimes become a source of hip pain. This condition is known as lateral hip pain, gluteal tendinopathy or trochanteric bursitis.

Functions of the hip region

The design of the hip supports our body weight and allows flexibility and strength for the performance of a range of physical tasks such as rising from sitting or putting on our socks (*Photo 13*) through to lifting and carrying heavy loads (*Photo 14*), walking, climbing or descending steps (*Photo 15*) and running (*Photo 16*).

Mechanical pain

Pain of mechanical origin occurs when a pain-sensitive structure is overstretched, overloaded or compressed, either by a single significant

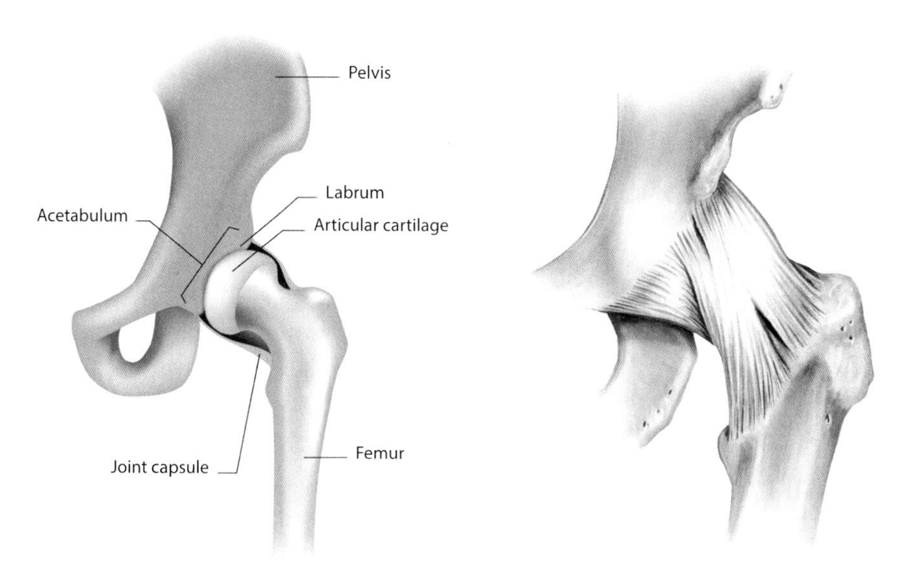

Figure 4 Pelvis and left hip

Figure 5 Hip capsule (left hip)

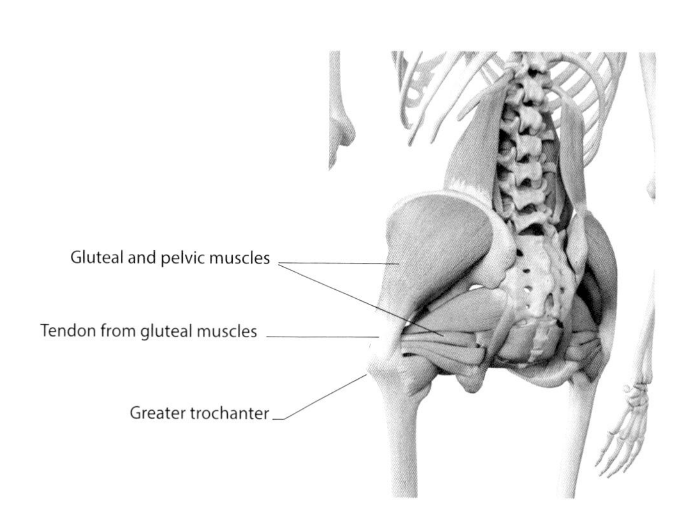

Figure 6 Lateral view of muscles (left hip)

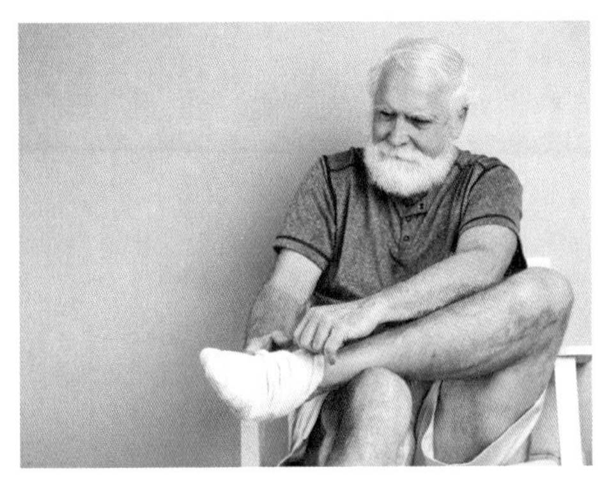

Photo 13 Putting on socks

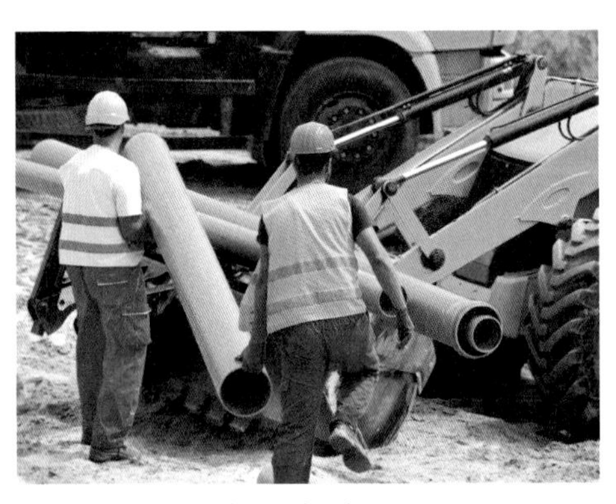

Photo 14 Carrying heavy loads

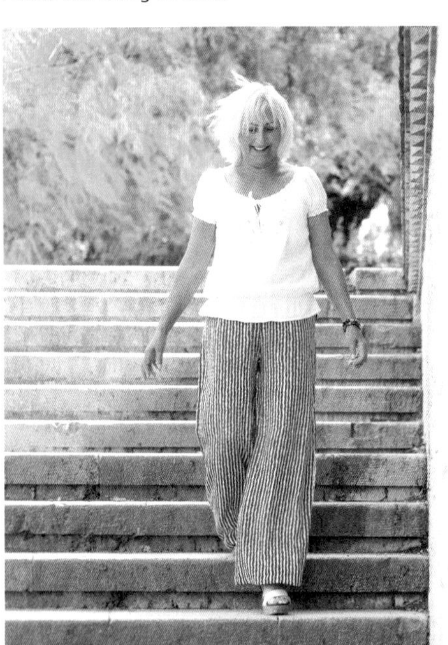

Photo 15 Walking down steps

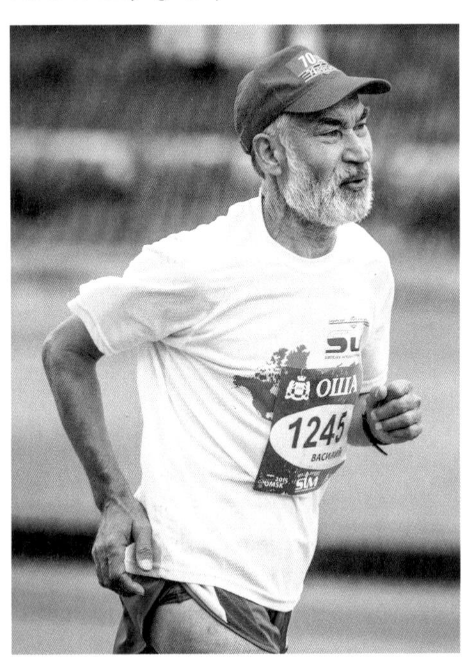

Photo 16 Running

event such as a fall or twist or repeated actions such as running downhill, or over a sustained duration such as prolonged standing. This is true for mechanical pain in any region of the body, including the hip. To help you understand how easily some mechanical pains can be produced, you may like to try a simple experiment. First, bend one finger backwards until you feel a strain, as shown in Photo 17.

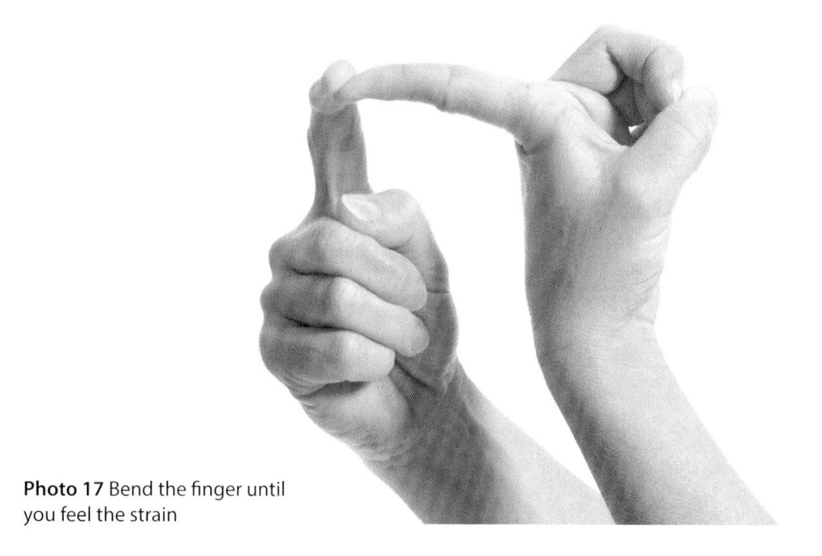

Photo 17 Bend the finger until you feel the strain

If you keep your finger in this position, you initially feel only minor discomfort, but as time passes, pain develops. In some cases, pain caused by prolonged stretching or compressive forces may take as much as an hour to be felt.

Try the experiment once more, but now keep bending the finger past the point of strain until you feel the immediate sensation of pain. You have overstretched, and your pain warning system is telling you that to continue movement in this particular direction will cause damage. The pain warning tells you to stop overstretching to avoid damage and, when you do so, the pain ceases immediately. No damage has occurred and the pain has gone. No lasting problems arise from this short-lived strain providing you take note of the pain warning system.

If you fail to heed the warning and keep the finger in the overstretched position, the ligaments and surrounding soft tissues that hold the joint together will eventually overstretch and tear.

This tearing will result in an ache that continues even when you stop overstretching. The discomfort or pain reduces in intensity but continues

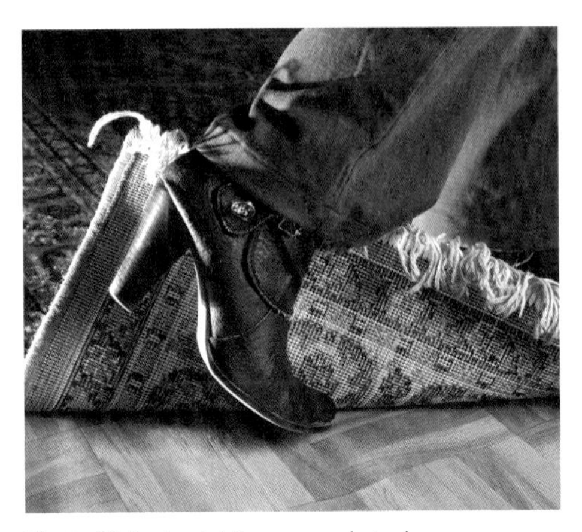

Photo 18 Foot catching on an obstacle

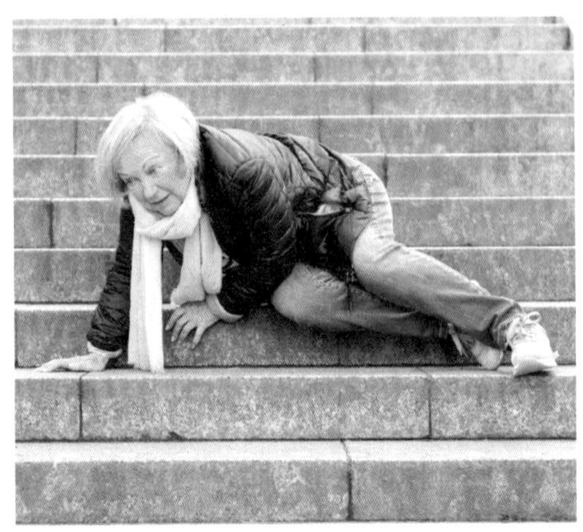

Photo 19 A fall onto the side of your hip

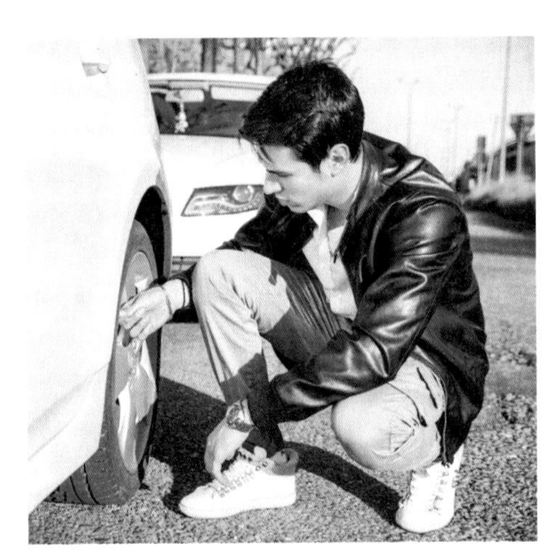

Photo 20 Sustained squatting

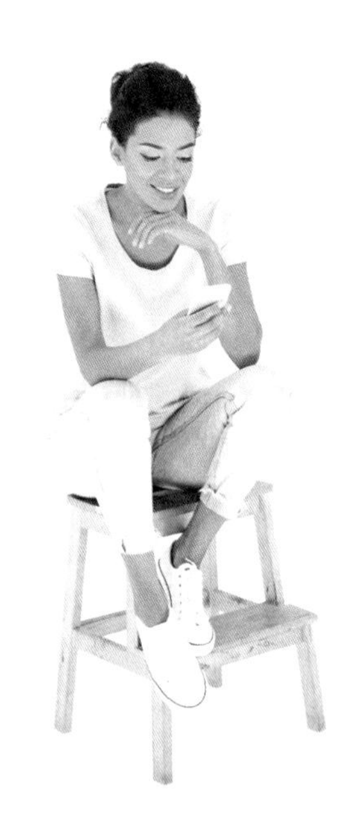

Photo 21 Sitting with hips bent more than 90 degrees

even when the finger is at rest. The pain increases when there is movement in the direction that has overstretched the affected tissues and will not cease until some healing has occurred. Healing may take several days, but would be prolonged if every day you were to continue to apply the same strains to the finger. The same things happen when you overstretch the structures in and around your hip.

Mechanical hip pain

In the hip region, the hip ligaments, capsule and surrounding tendons are responsible for supporting the hip joint and allowing movement to occur. Mechanical hip pain often arises due to overstretching, overloading or distorting these tissues. This may occur without further damage as in the bent finger example above. Overstretching may be caused by a force placing a sudden severe strain on the hip, for example a sudden twist when your foot catches on a step or obstacle (*Photo 18*) or a fall onto the side of your hip (*Photo 19*). This type of stress cannot easily be avoided as it occurs unexpectedly.

However, more often, overstretching or overloading is caused by postural stresses that place less severe strains on the hip over a longer time period. For example, performing work or activities where you are standing in the same position for a prolonged period of time, or performing an activity with either repeated or sustained bent hip positions such as squatting, for example changing a car tyre (*Photo 20*), or sitting with your hips bent more than 90 degrees (*Photo 21*). In some cases pain caused by prolonged standing or sitting may take as long as an hour to appear.

By understanding the potential for injury in repeatedly performing these actions or sustained static standing for prolonged periods of time, we can learn to minimise these adverse loads on our hips. Herein lies one of our main responsibilities in the self-treatment and prevention of hip pain.

Tissue damage

Complications arise when overstretching or overloading of soft tissues around the hip leads to actual tissue damage. It is often thought that hip pain is caused by strained muscles. This is not the case. Muscles, which are the source of power and movement, can be overstretched but usually heal rapidly and seldom cause pain lasting more than a week or two.

The real problem is the hip joint itself and its associated soft tissue structures which may be injured from overstretching or overloading. Pain from these injured structures will interfere with the normal function in the surrounding muscles, resulting in the muscles weakening. This further reduces the strength and function of the hip and makes the structures of the hip more vulnerable to further damage.

These damaged structures undergo a healing process that may result in an incomplete repair, and become less elastic and weakened. Once soft tissues are damaged, pain is felt until healing is complete and function is fully restored. In most cases, the solution for these pain-sensitive structures is to remodel the affected tissues by gradually applying progressive forces and avoiding or modifying the adverse loading on them. Unless appropriate exercises are performed to gradually stretch and strengthen these structures and restore their normal flexibility and function they will become a continuous source of hip pain. In frustration some people turn to medication or even surgery that may not be necessary.

NOTES

Chapter 3: Common causes of hip pain

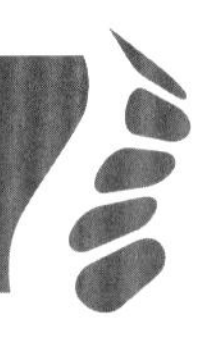

There are several structures within the hip region that can give rise to hip pain. These are the capsule and ligaments that hold the joint together, and the joint surfaces and underlying bone, which are the load-bearing components of the hip joint itself. There are also the tendons attaching the muscle groups from the pelvis to the outer aspect of the hip, as discussed in Chapter Two.

The hip is a very strong and stable joint, and acute traumatic injuries are far less common than those to the knee or ankle. However, it is still somewhat vulnerable to twisting forces or strains. Common events could be during sport (*Photo 22*), catching your foot or stepping in a hole and twisting your hip, or receiving a direct blow such as falling onto your hip (*Photo 23*), all of which can damage the joint surfaces, labrum or the ligaments or capsule (*Figures 4–6*).

If you are reading this book for the first time and have just injured your hip in this way within the last 24–48 hours, see the section on acute management in Chapter Six for information on how to manage a recent soft-tissue injury to the hip.

However, much more common than a specific injury or incident is hip pain that develops for no apparent reason. If we sustain static positions for long periods and only apply load sporadically through a small range of motion as is common in our adult lives, the hip joint gradually becomes less able to tolerate the peaks of load when we increase the loading on the hip too quickly. This can occur with a sudden increase in repetitive activities such as walking or running, or single actions that produce a sudden increased load on the hip such as a jump or deep squat.

It is this combination of normal aging changes, gradual deterioration of a healthy joint through lack of use, and associated injuries along the way that contribute to the development of hip pain, as the smooth cartilage erodes and other soft tissues become pain sensitive.

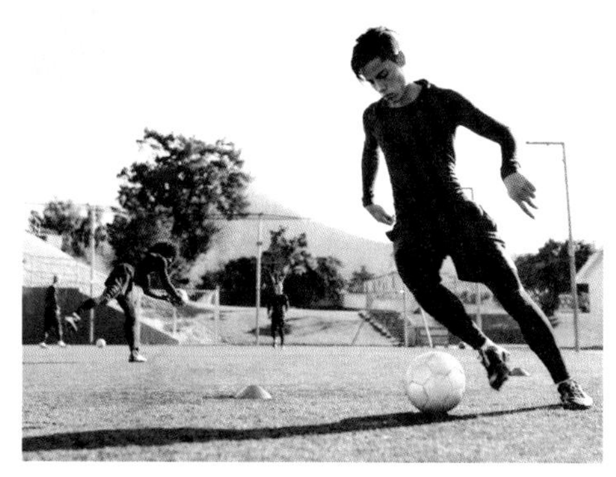

Photo 22 Twisting during sport

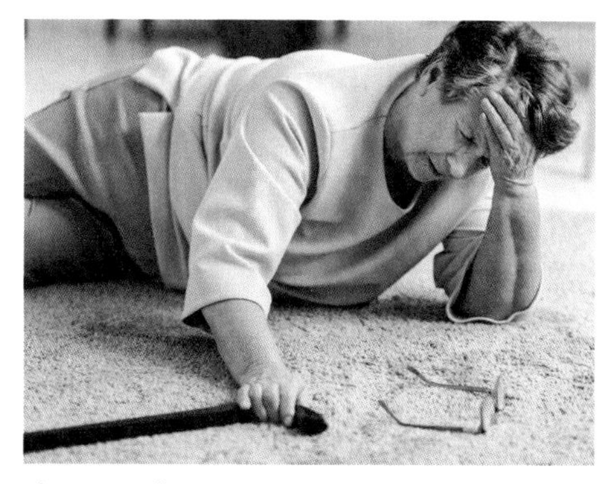

Photo 23 Falling onto your hip

If we lose the full range of painless motion and functional strength through the development of a painful hip, it quickly impacts on our daily life, and can affect everyday tasks such as dressing, drying your feet, walking or using stairs, or carrying heavy objects.

Like the other joints in the body, our hips require regular controlled movement and activity to nourish and maintain the structures in and around the hip to enable a high level of pain-free function.

Therefore, the most common issues that contribute to developing and prolonging hip pain relate to three main factors:

1. **Inactivity–low fitness levels**
2. **Postural stresses/prolonged standing or sitting**
3. **Being overweight**

1. Inactivity–low fitness levels

In our so-called 'modern' lifestyles, the great majority of us simply don't do enough general exercise for our hips. Our legs are designed for walking, running, climbing and jumping – but we spend little time doing these. Mostly, we fold our legs underneath us seated at a table or desk. Many of us have sedentary occupations where we sit most of the day, often at computers or driving (*Photo 24*). Then at home, most of us sit for prolonged periods in the evenings watching TV, eating a meal, or sitting at the computer. A 2010 study in Britain indicated that, on average, adults spend 14 hours a day sitting (*Photo 25*).

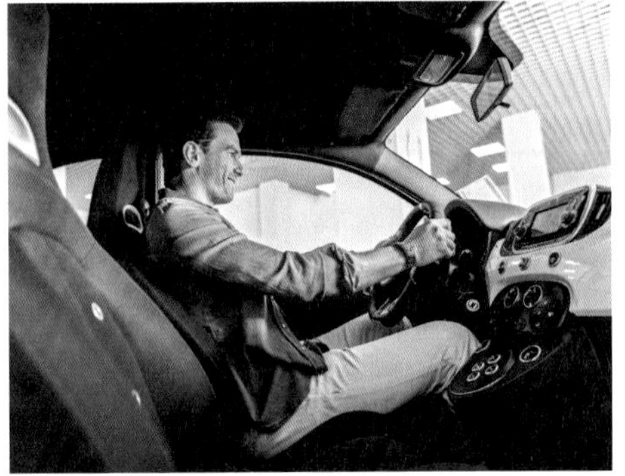

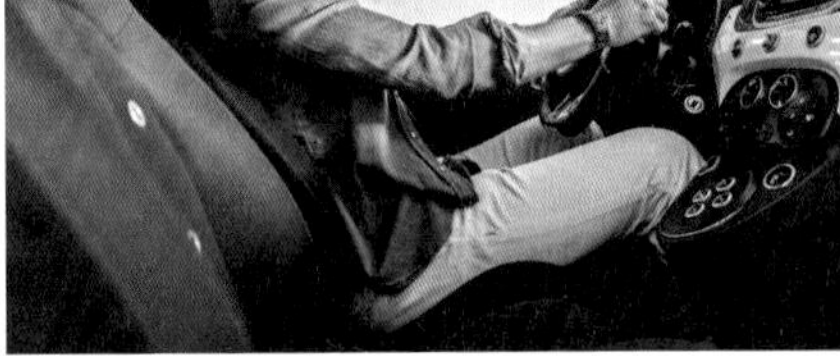

Photo 24 Prolonged driving

Photo 25 Prolonged sitting

It is no coincidence that many people develop recurrent and persisting hip pain in their forties and fifties. This is the stage of our lives when we gradually do less exercise, become more sedentary, and it is also the stage when our body's metabolism changes and we have a tendency to put on weight. Additionally it is the age when the tissues of the body begin to become less flexible and lose the capacity to absorb adverse load. Between the ages of 50 and 70, we lose about 30 per cent of our strength from disuse. The average 20-year-old uses 20 per cent of their capacity to rise from a chair; the average 70-year-old uses 90 per cent. Often hip pain causes avoidance of activities which would strengthen the legs, such as walking or stair climbing.

Think back to when you were a child, and remember how active you once were, or simply observe a group of children. It is difficult for them to sit for any length of time; their natural inclination is to be on the move. Then, when they do get up, what do they do? They invariably run around, or hop, jump or skip. All the time they are using the joints and muscles of their legs, and developing the endurance and strength to perform increasing amounts of sustained physical activity.

Contrast this to adults. It is unusual for us to be on the move for any length of time, and our natural inclination is to get back to sitting as soon as possible. What do you do in your lunch break at work after sitting all morning? Most likely you walk a few steps and then sit again for the majority of your break. Similarly, our city and urban communities, with shopping malls and public buildings, provide us with all sorts of

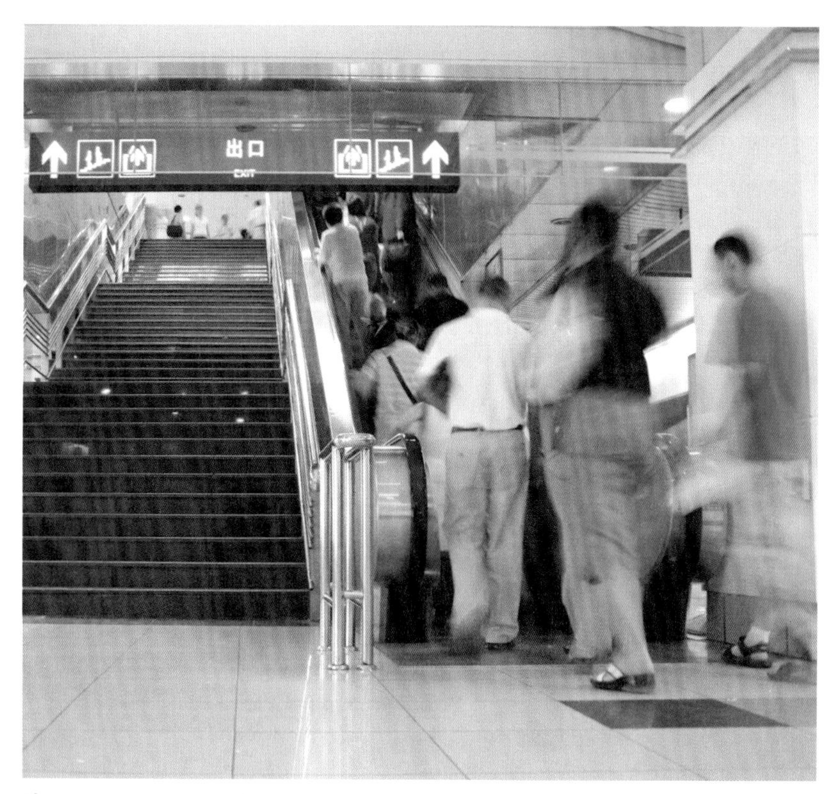

Photo 26 Using an escalator instead of the stairs

facilities that minimise the amount of walking we have to do. We drive our cars or take public transport as close as possible to our destination, we use escalators or elevators (*Photo 26*), and we sit on the available stools, benches or chairs provided at every opportunity.

This less-physical lifestyle results in reduced activity levels, and as our fitness declines further, our body weight and the corresponding load on the hips tend to increase.

The hip joint and its surrounding muscles respond to appropriate exercise and load. Regularly loading the hip with physical activity assists with the nutrition within the hip and keeps the surrounding muscles flexible and strong, which in turn maintains the hip's sense of balance and co-ordination. Conversely, if we don't keep active we don't put our hips through a full range of movement, and they gradually lose range of motion. This contributes to loss of muscle strength and a decrease in our tolerance to perform sustained levels of physical activity. This contributes to mechanical pain, as well as making our hips more susceptible to sudden twisting or impact stresses described at the start of this chapter.

However, there is very good evidence in the medical literature for increasing our general activity to reverse this decline in the strength and function of our hips. Also, many studies have shown that this 'training' effect on the body's tissues occurs even well into older age if the loading is graduated and regular. It is never too late to get more active providing you start gently.

Chapter Six describes simple ideas and effective strategies to assist you with a graduated increase in your activities to improve and maintain your hip function.

Regularly loading our hips with appropriate physical activity assists with the nutrition within our hips and keeps the surrounding muscle groups flexible and strong, which in turn increases our hips' ability to perform daily activities.

---

2. Postural stresses

As well as problems caused by inactivity, there are some specific hip positions that contribute to excess stress on the joint structures. These stresses arise from prolonged or repeated activities which can adversely load the hip-joint structures.

These are primarily a combination of three factors:

- Standing still for extended periods of time places a prolonged static load through the hip-joint surfaces without giving them time to recover in an unloaded position. Standing for prolonged periods with the majority of your body weight through one leg will increase the adverse load through that hip region.
- Lying and sleeping with a painful hip positioned incorrectly can place either direct pressure or an inappropriate postural stress on the affected structures of the hip.

- Performing repetitive or prolonged tasks with our hips bent, while taking some load through the hip, for example, prolonged crouching without taking regular breaks from this position, or prolonged sitting with bent hips, in a low chair.

Postural neglect

When these postures are maintained long enough, they cause overstretching or overloading of the structures in and around the hip. Thus pain will arise only in certain positions. Hip problems developed in this way are the *consequence of postural neglect.* Sustained hip posture is not the only cause of hip pain. However, once hip problems have developed, sustained postures will frequently make them worse and perpetuate them.

Some people who habitually adopt poor hip postures and remain unaware of the underlying cause experience hip pain throughout their adult lifetime simply because they didn't receive the necessary information to correct the postural faults.

Pains of postural origin are often first felt as a minor irritation and are easily ignored as they are eliminated merely by correcting the postures. However, as time passes, these uncorrected habitual hip postures cause changes to the structures of the hip. Excessive wear occurs, with loss of elasticity resulting in degenerative changes to the structures in and around the hip. Pain becomes more frequent and persistent.

The effects of poor posture and general inactivity in the long term, therefore, can be just as severe and harmful as the effects of injury.

Should pain develop, there are certain movements or posture modifications you can perform in order to stop that pain. You should *not* have to seek assistance whenever postural pain arises.

Prolonged sitting postures

You may have been sitting with bent hips for many years without hip pain. However, consistently sitting with your hip bent in one position for a period of time, for example at a cramped work station, will gradually cause an overstretching and overloading of the structures in and around the hip. You will often find your hip is initially stiff and uncomfortable as

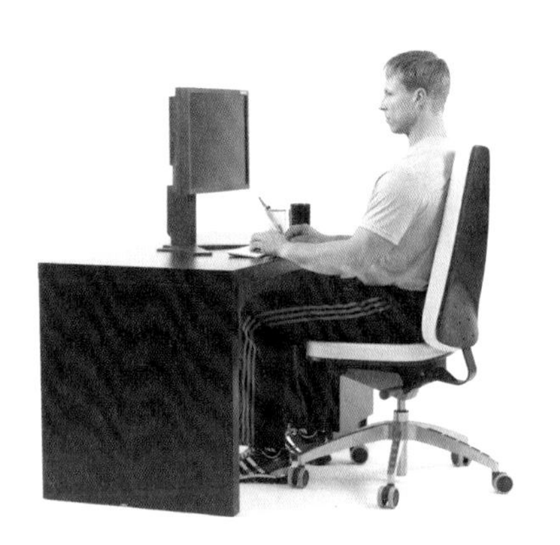

Photo 27 Sitting with hips bent less than 90 degrees

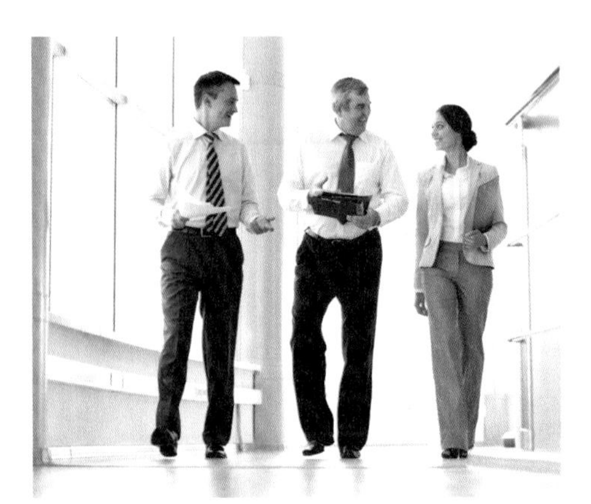

Photo 28 Going for a short walk

you stand up from the prolonged sitting position, and take the first few steps. If you continue to persist with the static, bent hip posture your hip will become painful in the sitting position as well as when you rise from sitting. If you already have hip pain you will have probably noticed how bent hip-sitting aggravates your pain.

How to manage prolonged sitting

If your hip pain is either produced or aggravated by prolonged sitting, it is important to correct the posture causing the pain. It is also necessary to take a regular break from your activity to stand up and go for a short walk. As a general rule avoid sitting with your hip bent more than 90 degrees (*Photo 27*), and if more comfortable use a low foot stool as recommended in good work-space design. At every refreshment break ensure you go for a walk of at least a few minutes to allow your hip to recover from being bent up in one position. Further strategies to assist with interrupting prolonged sitting are discussed in Chapter Six on pages 77 and 78.

Prolonged standing postures

When you stand in one position for long enough your affected hip will start to feel uncomfortable from the static loading you are placing through the joint. You may take a few steps to ease the discomfort but the pain will return once you return to a static standing position again. If you are standing on a concrete floor or wearing footwear without cushioning soles, the onset of hip pain is likely to occur sooner.

As time passes this sustained standing in one position can cause changes to the weight-bearing structures within the hip. The joint surfaces will lose their shock-absorbing capacity and become painful when you are standing for any duration.

How to manage prolonged standing

If you have developed hip pain from standing still for prolonged periods, it is necessary for you to remove this adverse postural stress on your hip by either sitting briefly or going for a short walk every 30 minutes (*Photo 28*). Both are ways of altering the static load through the hip.

At each refreshment break, go for a short walk, or if that is not possible 'march on the spot' in order to alter the loading on your hip. If your hip pain continues you will find it necessary to sit on a chair or stool to unload your hip.

Prolonged standing on a concrete floor places more stress on the hip than standing on a wooden floor. Supportive footwear with cushioned soles will also assist in reducing the adverse load being placed through your hips, as well as standing on cushioning mats.

Lying and sleeping

If you wake up in the morning with a painful hip that was not causing problems the night before, or your hip pain wakes you consistently during the night, it is likely there is something wrong with the position of your hip when you sleep. If you are lying in a position that is placing an adverse stress on your hip, either by lying on your side with your hips pressed together or lying with your hip in a fully extended or bent position, a gradual overloading or overstretching of the painful structures occurs. Thus poor sleeping postures can further aggravate an already painful hip.

How to manage sleeping and lying

There are two things to consider with hip pain from lying or sleeping. If you lie on your painful side this will place a compressive load and often can only be tolerated for a short period before you have to change position. Many people find lying on their non-painful side (*Photo 29*) with a pillow between their knees takes some of the load off the affected hip. It is also necessary to avoid lying with your affected hip either bent up past 90 degrees or fully straightened out as these positions will place

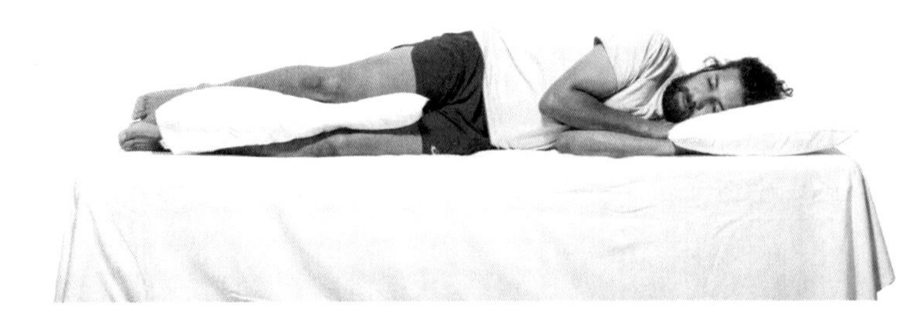

Photo 29 Lying on non-painful side with pillow between legs

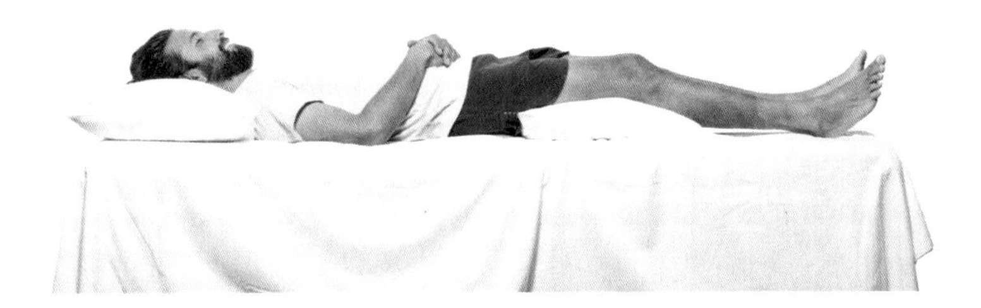

Photo 30 Lying on back with pillow under knees

adverse postural stresses on your hip. If this does not provide relief, it is recommended you sleep on your back with a pillow under your knees (*Photo 30*) to provide support as this also avoids placing your hip in the fully extended position.

3. Being overweight

Many groups such as the Osteoarthritis Research Society International and the National Institute of Health and Clinical Excellence in UK clearly link being overweight to the onset of hip pain in adults. Many of us gradually put on excess weight through our middle years – again, mostly as a result of our modern lifestyle. But we also find it harder at this stage of our lives to find the time and the desire to exercise sufficiently.

A moderate loss of weight results in a significant decrease in loading on the hip, and in most cases a 5 per cent loss in weight would be a reasonable target for which to aim.

A commonly used formula to approximately measure the percentage of body fat is the Body Mass Index or BMI. It is defined as an individual's body weight divided by the square of his or her height, and an average BMI is approximately 20–30 (kg/m^2). Numerous studies have confirmed that having a BMI over 25 points is associated with increased risk of hip pain and associated loss of function. There is also an increased likelihood of developing other health problems such as diabetes, high blood pressure, heart attacks and a shortened lifespan. It is easy to measure your BMI to determine whether you are overweight. An online search will also show a number of websites that do the calculation for you once you enter your height, weight and age.

The American Academy of Orthopaedic Surgeons also identifies 25 as an appropriate baseline, and recommends 5 per cent weight loss for anybody with a BMI greater than 25 if OA changes are evident on an X-ray (that is most of us in our forties and fifties and above). It has shown that a modest loss in weight results in a significant decrease in hip pain, and in most cases 5 per cent would appear to be a reasonable target to aim for. For many people this can be achieved over a few weeks or months by eating less or differently with an appropriate weight loss regime, and exercising more. Some simple advice and strategies for losing weight and increasing general exercise are covered further in Chapter Six. However, we recommend you seek advice from your doctor or physician, or attend a recognised weight-loss programme, should you have underlying health issues or seek to lose a significant amount of weight.

Lateral hip pain

One relatively common and frustrating source of hip pain is pain felt only at the outside (lateral region) of the hip. One hip is usually affected but sometimes both hips will be affected to some extent.

This painful condition is generally called lateral hip pain because of the uncertainty about a specific cause, and therefore there is also uncertainty about the best treatment options. Variations of the condition are also referred to as trochanteric bursitis, tendinitis, or gluteal tendinopathy. Generally it is recognised that excessive repetitive forces on the hip joint region can affect the load on the lateral hip structures statically or dynamically and cause adverse load through these lateral tissues.

The factors causing lateral hip pain are not fully understood, but losing the flexibility, strength and co-ordination in the muscles around the hip can all be contributing factors. The condition frequently affects endurance sports people such as runners or cyclists, people in their forties and fifties, and women more than men, particularly if overweight, and the problem may continue for many years. Often lateral hip pain comes on for no apparent reason, but sometimes it is associated with a sudden increase in a new activity, such as a sport that involves sudden changes in direction or jumping, or hiking in hill country. A fall onto the side of the hip or prolonged standing may also trigger lateral hip pain.

People with lateral hip pain frequently find one hip has a full range of motion with no obstruction to movement compared to the other leg. The pain is usually produced or made worse with prolonged standing with one hip taking more weight, carrying a heavy weight regularly on that side, performing an aggravating activity such as walking down stairs or hills, or playing a chosen sport.

Conventional treatments often have a lack of long-term success and therefore the emphasis needs to be placed on the person to apply effective ongoing self-treatment.

The information regarding appropriate hip positions and activity modifications in this chapter will be important in minimising and managing your lateral hip pain. Chapter 5 (page 54) will explain how to determine if your lateral hip pain will benefit from the treatment described in this book, and give guidance as to when to seek further advice from a health care professional.

Ongoing pain and reduced function following hip surgery

While hip joint replacement surgery is regarded as one of the most successful orthopaedic procedures, there are a group of people who have had hip surgery, including replacements, who continue to have hip pain and difficulty walking, climbing stairs or performing their daily activities. The treatment options for this group are discussed in Chapter 5.

NOTES

Chapter 4: Understanding the McKenzie Method®

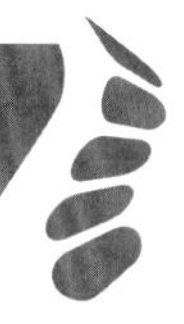

The aim of the exercises

The aim of the exercises is to abolish pain and, where appropriate, to restore normal function – that is, to regain full mobility and strength in the hip or as much movement as possible under the given circumstances.

When you are exercising for **pain relief**, you should move **just into the pain**, then release the pressure and return to the starting position. As you release the stretch, the pain must diminish back to the starting level or less. If it does not, you are overdoing it, and must use less force on your next attempt. When you are exercising for **stiffness**, the exercises can be made more effective by firmly and steadily applying 'overpressure', as described in Chapter Five (page 63), in order to obtain the maximum amount of movement. In this case a feeling of discomfort may persist afterwards but not for more than 20 minutes, otherwise you are overdoing it and need to apply less pressure next time.

Always try and maintain correct hip postures and positions following the exercises. Once you no longer have hip pain, ongoing good postural habits are essential to prevent the recurrence of hip pain.

Effect on pain intensity and location

There are three main effects to look for while performing the exercises:

1. **They may cause the symptoms to disappear.**
2. **They may cause an increase or decrease in the intensity of the pain that you experience.**
3. **They may cause the pain to move from where you usually feel it to some other location.**

In certain cases the symptoms first change location, then they reduce in intensity and finally they cease altogether.

The effects of exercise on intensity or location of pain can sometimes be very rapid. It is possible to reduce the intensity or change the location of pain after completing as few as ten movements, and in some conditions the pain can completely disappear.

In order to determine whether the exercise programme is beneficial for you, it is important that you observe closely any changes in the location of the pain. You may notice that pain, originally felt on the front or outside side of your hip, or groin, moves to a different location in your hip as a result of the exercises.

Pain intensity

If your hip pain is of such intensity that you can only move your leg with difficulty and cannot find a position to lie comfortably in bed, your approach to the exercises should be cautious and unhurried.

On commencing any of the exercises you may experience an initial increase in pain. This is common and can be expected. As you continue to practise, the pain should quickly diminish, at least to its former level. Usually this occurs during the first exercise session. This will often be followed by the pain becoming more localised to one area of the hip joint. Once the pain becomes localised, the intensity of the pain will generally steadily decrease over a period of a few days and by continuing the exercises, the pain will often disappear entirely.

However, if following an initial pain increase, the pain continues to increase in intensity or spreads to places further away from the hip such as the thigh or the knee, you should stop exercising and seek advice. In other words, do not continue with any of the exercises if your symptoms are much worse immediately after exercising and **remain worse the next day**; or if during exercising, symptoms are produced or increased further down your leg.

As discussed earlier, once you have started this exercise programme, you should expect new exercise pains to develop. These are different from your original pain and are usually felt in areas of the hip which were previously not affected. New pains are the result of performing work your body is not used to and, provided you continue with the exercises, they will wear off in three to four days.

If your symptoms have been present continuously for many weeks or months, you should not expect to be pain-free in two to three days. The response will be slower, but, if you are doing the correct exercises, it will only be a matter of time before the pain subsides.

As long as your pain is slowly improving, continue with the exercise programme. Do not change anything in your newly established routine, including no change to pain medication at first. It may be tempting to add other exercises, but this may disrupt your progress. Wait until improvement stops or your pain is 75 per cent better before progressing your exercise programme, or considering a cautious start with any other activity or exercise.

Starting the exercise programme

When you commence this exercise programme you should stop any other exercise that you may have been shown elsewhere or you happen to do regularly, for example, for fitness or sport. If you want to continue with exercises other than the ones described in this book for hip problems, you should wait until your pains have subsided completely.

NOTES

Chapter 5: The exercise programme

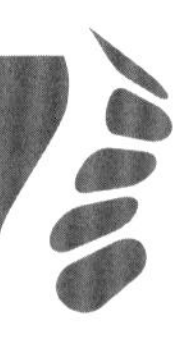

Overview

In the opening chapters we have outlined the conditions that can cause pain, reduce mobility and limit function in your hip. As discussed in Chapter One (pages 12 and 13), it is sometimes difficult to determine exactly what hip condition you have, and therefore which exercises to perform.

It is vital to follow the exercise sequence outlined in this chapter as it is a systematic approach that will enable you to successfully self-treat your hip condition.

This chapter describes and clearly illustrates a series of exercises, and also gives you information as to **when** to apply the exercises and the responses to expect.

We recommend you try each of the following five exercises first with your non-painful leg, and then cautiously attempt the same exercise with your painful leg. In this way you can compare the pain and range of motion in both hips and use this as a baseline to monitor your progress as you perform the programme to reduce the pain, and restore the mobility and function in your painful hip.

If you are in significant pain

If you have an acute flare up of your hip pain, or this is a recent injury, we recommend you review the question on page 18 in Chapter One: 'Is the information in this book suitable for me?' If none of the situations described relate to you, we recommend you refer to the section on Acute Management on page 74 in Chapter Six before commencing this programme.

It is also important when you have hip pain to follow the postural education in Chapter Three (page 42) in an attempt to find resting positions where you are as comfortable as possible in sitting, standing and lying.

When your pain reduces or you are able to walk more comfortably you can commence the exercise programme.

When acute or severe pain has subsided

When significant pain has subsided or you have only intermittent pain you may still feel some pain when moving your hip in certain ways. You will notice this when attempting activities such as walking, using stairs or running or when you are required to bend your hip such as sitting, crouching, putting on your socks, lifting an object from the ground or sitting cross-legged. It is likely there is an obstruction to movement within your hip or your hip has stiffened up over a period of time following damage to the tissues around the hip or to the joint surfaces of the hip joint.

The aim of the structured exercise sequence outlined below is to reduce your pain and restore the flexibility and function to your affected hip without causing further damage.

Exercises 1 to 3 will assist with reducing and often abolishing your hip pain, and will also improve hip range of motion and function. Exercises 4 and 5 will assist with restoring strength and endurance in the surrounding muscles when your hip has a normal range of motion yet is still painful, and they can also be used effectively to treat a condition called lateral hip pain, known as trochanteric bursitis or gluteal tendinopathy.

To start this process of recovery

Exercises 1–3 will help reduce then abolish the pain in your hip and groin region.

Commence with Exercise 1: Hip extension in kneeling.

Exercise 1: Hip extension in kneeling

This exercise helps reduce then abolish the pain in your hip and groin region and assists in restoring the ability of your hip to perform daily activities such as walking and going up and down stairs or crouching/squatting.

Place a chair beside you to assist with balance, and a folded towel or small cushion under your knee for comfort. Start by half-kneeling, with the knee of your affected hip on the towel or cushion and your unaffected leg in front of you. (*Photo 31*). Ensure that your affected leg is pointing directly behind you (*Photo 32*). Place your hand behind your affected hip. Let your affected hip relax. Slowly lunge forward, keeping your body

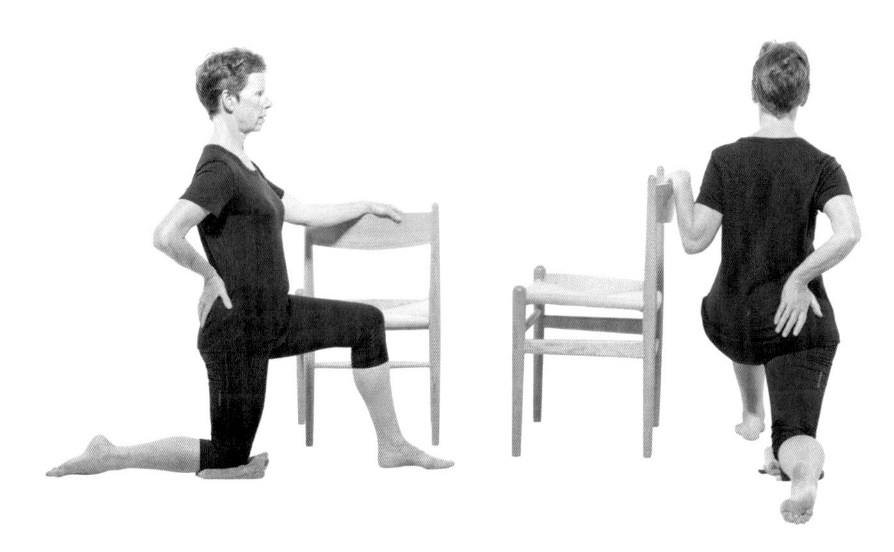

Photo 31 Starting position with chair for support

Photo 32 Affected leg pointing directly behind

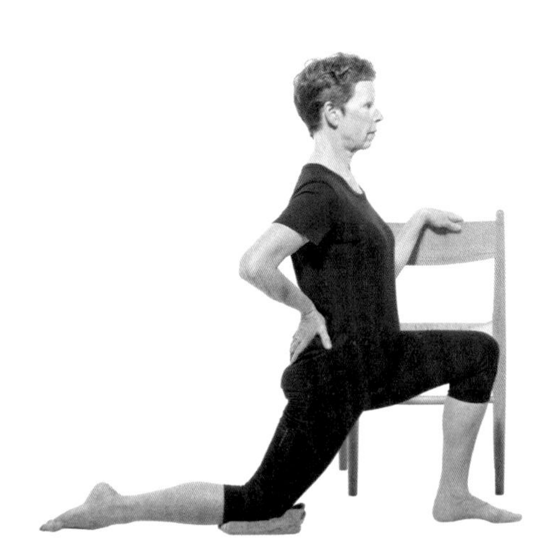

Photo 33 Hip extension in kneeling

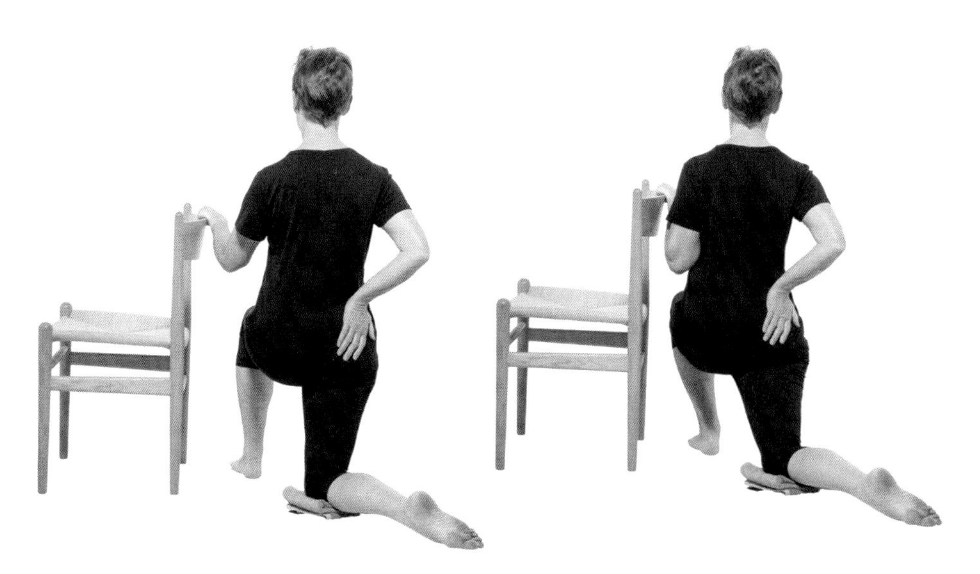

Photo 34 Hip extension in kneeling with internal rotation

Photo 35 Push your hip forward with your hand

upright while also applying a forward pressure with your hand behind your affected hip until you feel a firm stretch on the front of your affected hip (*Photo 33*).

Hold for a few seconds and then return your hip to the starting position. Each time you perform this movement, try to slowly lunge forward a little further so that by the end of 10 repetitions, you have reached your maximum possible hip extension.

Exercise 1 should be repeated 10 times per session and the sessions should be spread evenly four to six times throughout the day until bed time. This means you should repeat the sessions about every two to three hours.

Over a few days you should find your hip pain reduces or is more localised and there is improved movement. You should also be able to progress this exercise to ensure you are getting to end range by pushing your hip forward more firmly with your hand.

If your hip has stopped improving with this exercise it is necessary to progress Exercise 1 by performing the exercise with your affected rear leg turned outwards to add an internal rotation stretch to your hip (*Photos 34 and 35*). Ensure you are using a chair for support.

Again, this variation of Exercise 1 should be repeated ten times per session and the sessions should be spread evenly four to six times throughout the day until you go to bed at night. This means you should repeat the sessions about every two to three hours.

Review your progress

If you find your hip pain is reducing or localising, and your movement and function has increased after performing Exercise 1, continue this exercise for a further two to six weeks, gradually lessening the number of times a day until your hip is non-painful.

Pain is often rapidly improved as you gain more movement inside the hip. However, stiffness rather than pain is more due to shortened tissue around the hip joint, which must gradually be lengthened over a longer period of time.

Once your hip is non-painful, or you have only occasional residual discomfort, perform Exercises 2 and 3 to restore the normal range of flexion and rotation to your affected hip to enable you to perform activities such as putting on your socks or crossing your legs.

The rule is to always finish with the exercise that corrected the initial painful problem, therefore perform Exercise 1 once you have completed Exercise 2 or 3.

Exercise 2: Hip flexion in sitting

This exercise helps in restoring the ability of your hip to perform daily activities such as going up and down stairs or crouching/squatting.

Sit upright in a firm chair (*Photo 36*). If you sit forward on the edge of the chair and lean back you will find it easier to perform this exercise. Slowly bend your affected hip up towards you, and with both hands pull up on your leg just below your knee. Slowly pull your knee towards your chest until you feel a firm tension at your hip (*Photo 37*). Bring your knee as close as possible to your chest, and hold for a few seconds, then return your knee to the starting position. You may need to lean further back to achieve maximum effect (*Photo 38*). Each time you perform this movement cycle, try to bend your hip a little further, until you have reached the maximum possible flexion over 10 repetitions.

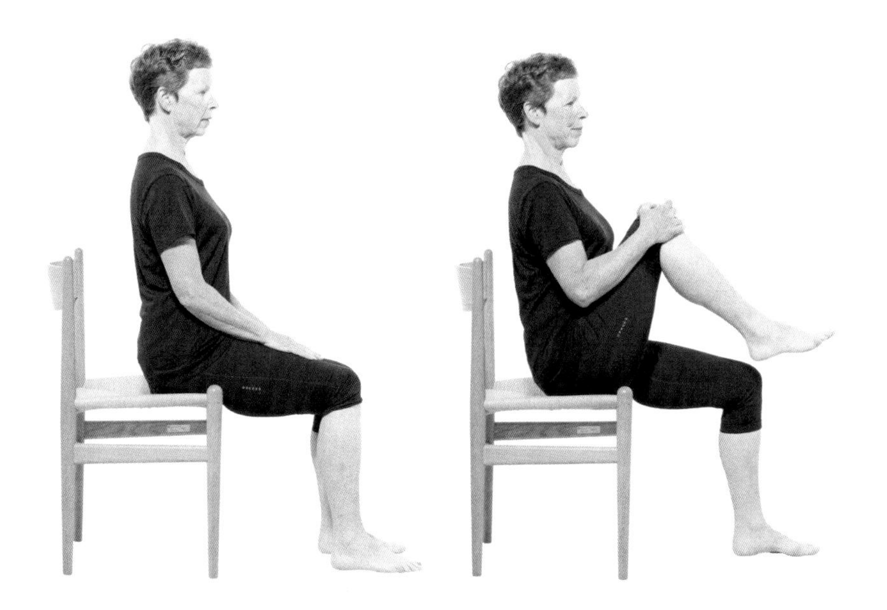

Photo 36 Sitting in chair

Photo 37 Hip flexion in sitting

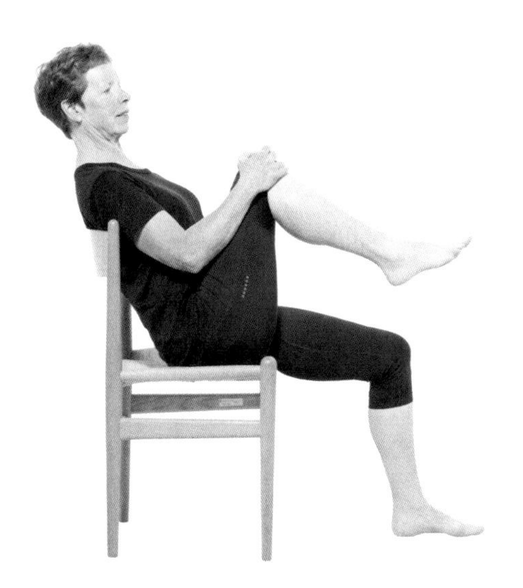

Photo 38 Lean back further for maximum effect

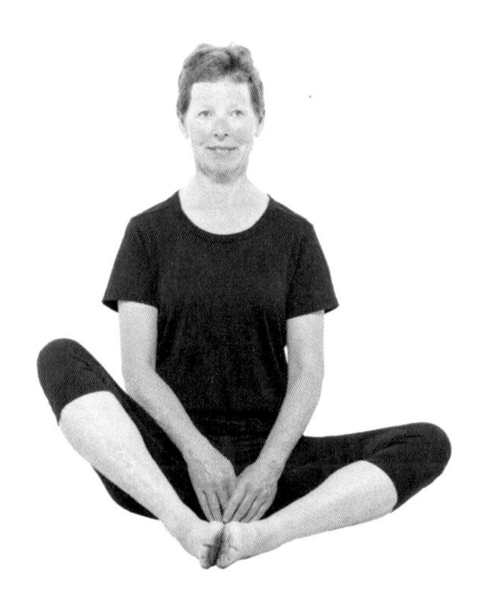

Photo 39 Sitting with back against wall

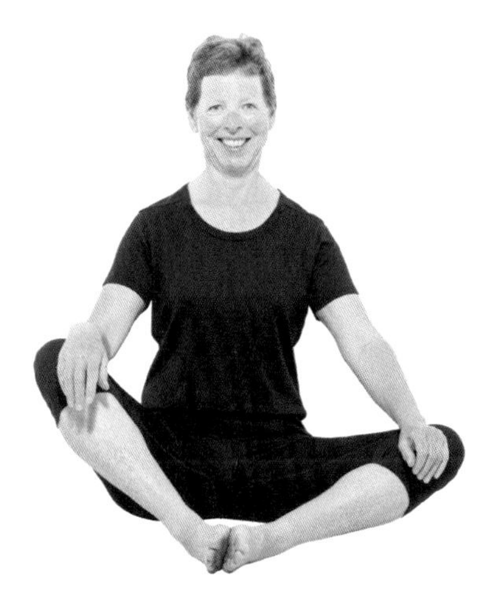

Photo 40 Apply downward pressure on your legs

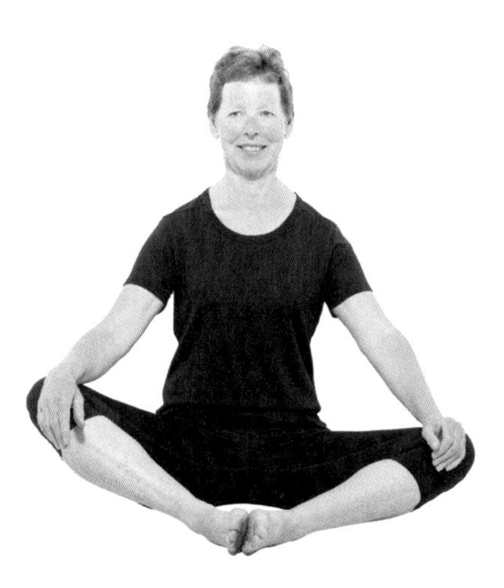

Photo 41 Try to allow your affected leg to stretch closer to the floor

Exercise 2 should be repeated 10 times per session and the sessions should be spread evenly four to six times throughout the day until bed time. This means you should repeat the sessions about every two to three hours.

Exercise 3: Hip abduction and external rotation in sitting

This exercise is used to restore the ability of your affected hip to enable you to sit cross-legged or perform activities such as drying your feet. Two options are described. If getting down into a sitting position on the floor is too difficult, choose the alternative position described below: sitting in a chair.

Sit on the floor with your back against a wall, bend your hips and knees and bring the soles of your feet together allowing your knees to move outwards (*Photo 39*). You may notice that the knee of your affected hip is higher off the ground than your unaffected side. This indicates your affected hip has a loss of external rotation. Place your forearms or hands on the insides of your shins (*Photo 40*). Relax your hips and allow them to reach the maximum possible external rotation, then slowly push downwards on your shins with your forearms or hands until you feel a firm stretch at your affected hip (*Photo 41*). Once you have held this position for a few seconds release the pressure and return to the starting position. Repeat the exercise 10 times. Each time you perform this movement cycle try to relax your leg and allow your affected leg to stretch closer to the floor until you have reached the maximum possible abduction and external rotation.

Exercise 3 should be repeated 10 times per session and the sessions should be spread evenly four to six times throughout the day until bed time. This means you should repeat the sessions about every two to three hours.

Alternative: sitting position in a chair

Sit on a chair with both feet flat on the floor. Try this exercise with the unaffected leg first. Lift the unaffected leg, bend your hip and knee and bring your foot onto your opposite thigh just above the knee. Allow your knee to move outwards (*Photo 42*). Return the leg to the starting position and repeat the exercise with the affected leg (*Photo 43*). You may notice that the knee of your affected hip is higher and more uncomfortable compared to your unaffected side. This indicates your affected hip has a loss of external rotation. Place your hand on the inside of your knee. Relax your hip and allow it to reach the maximum possible external rotation,

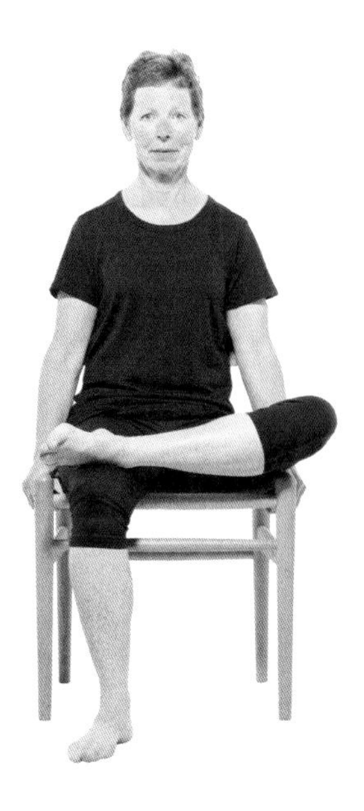

Photo 42 Try this exercise first with your unaffected leg

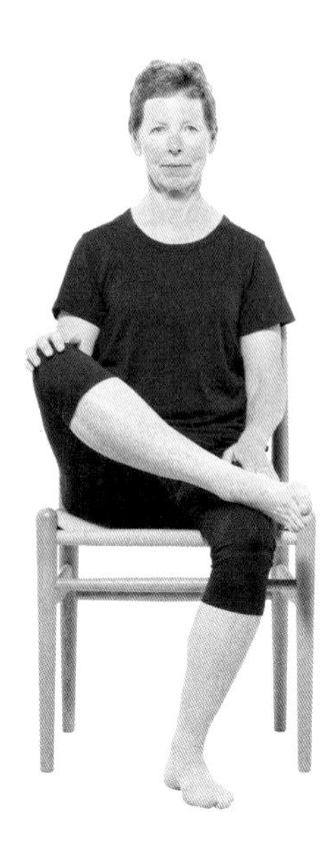

Photo 43 Then try the exercise with your affected leg

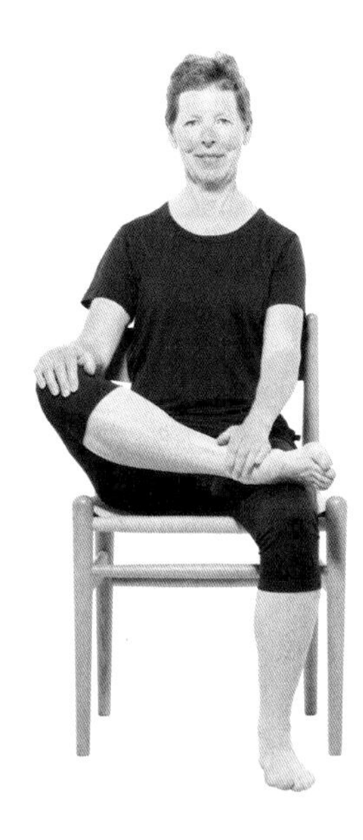

Photo 44 Apply downward pressure on your affected leg

then slowly push downwards on your knee with your hand until you feel a firm stretch at your affected hip (*Photo 44*). Once you have held this position for a few seconds release the pressure and return to the starting position. Repeat the exercise 10 times. Each time you perform this movement cycle try to relax your leg and allow your affected leg to stretch closer to the floor until you have reached the maximum possible abduction and external rotation.

Exercise 3 should be repeated 10 times per session and the sessions should be spread evenly four to six times throughout the day until bed time. This means you should repeat the sessions about every two to three hours.

Review your progress

If you feel only stiffness rather than pain on performing Exercise 2 or Exercise or 3, continue to perform these exercises, applying more overpressure at the end of each movement. By exercising in this way you achieve movement to the maximum degree. In most cases you will restore normal function within six weeks.

However, if you have found that either Exercise 2 or Exercise 3 increases your hip pain, discontinue with these exercises and continue with Exercise 1 as this is the exercise that has reduced your pain.

Once you have restored the normal range of motion to your affected hip and are able to perform Exercises 1 to 3 fully, with no pain, you will usually find no hip pain continues and you have regained the functional use of your affected hip.

However, do not forget the important postural education in Chapter Three (page 42) to prevent the onset of hip pain at rest.

When you are symptom-free follow the guidelines under the heading: **When you have no pain or stiffness** on page 68, to prevent recurrence of hip problems.

No response or benefit

If, after performing Exercises 1 to 3 for a few weeks, you still experience hip pain on activities such as prolonged standing or walking up or down stairs or hills, it is necessary to strengthen the ligaments, muscles and tendons around your hip. Progress to Exercise 4 and Exercise 5.

Lateral hip pain

As described earlier in Chapter Three on page 47, lateral hip pain is one of the conditions that can be challenging to treat successfully, and requires a programme of carefully performed exercises to achieve a successful outcome. If you continue to experience lateral hip pain we recommend you first perform Exercises 1 to 3, to ensure your hip is moving freely and that a loss of movement is not the underlying cause of the pain.

Exercises 4 and 5 are designed to reduce your lateral hip pain and increase the weight-bearing capacity and function of the injured tendons around your hip in order to perform daily activities more easily. Start cautiously with a few repetitions through a small range of motion, and gradually increase the number of repetitions. You may feel some discomfort in the muscles around your hip initially, which is to be expected but this should not worsen as you repeat these exercises.

Any pain produced from performing these exercises should go away within 15 minutes of completing the exercise session. If not, you are exercising too vigorously. If you have access to a swimming pool Exercises 4 and 5 can also be performed in waist-deep water initially.

Exercise 4: Hip strengthening – hip abduction in standing

Abduction means pushing your leg sideways away from the body. This exercise strengthens the gluteal muscles and tendons around the hip.

Stand facing a table or back of a chair, and support yourself with your fingers or hands as much as required (*Photo 45*). Slowly lift the leg of your painful hip sideways. Check the heel of your affected leg is turned outwards during the movement to ensure the exercise is performed correctly (*Photo 46*). Hold this position for three seconds then return to the starting position. Each time you perform this movement cycle try to emphasise pushing outwards with your heel so you feel a firm tension with some minor discomfort on the outer aspect of your hip during each repetition of the exercise. However, any discomfort produced must settle within 15 minutes of completing each set of 10 repetitions.

When used in the treatment of lateral hip pain or hip pain that has not responded to Exercises 1 to 3, Exercise 4 should be repeated 10 times per session and sessions should be repeated two times a day – once in the morning and once in the afternoon or evening.

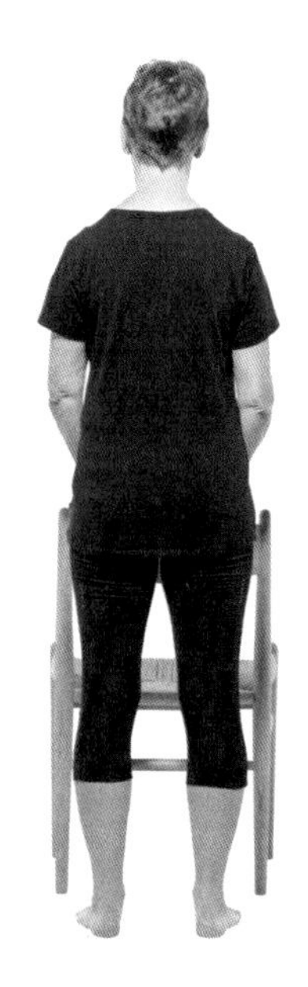

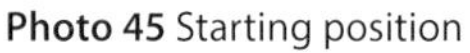

Photo 45 Starting position

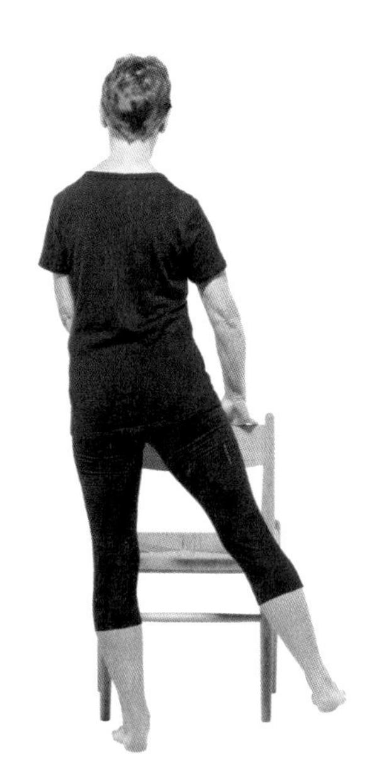

Photo 46 Hip abduction in standing– affected leg out to side

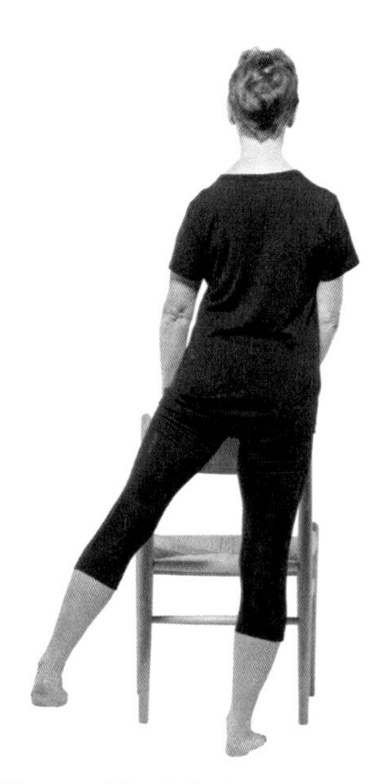

Photo 47 Hip abduction in standing – unaffected leg out to side

NOTE: This exercise can be performed in two ways. Once you are confident with the exercise above you can also try standing on your affected leg, and lifting the unaffected leg as a progression. This ensures the muscles around your affected hip are working to maintain your balance. Stand as above, taking minimal weight through your fingers or hands on a stable surface, and slowly lift your unaffected leg out to the side (*Photo 47*). Start with a few repetitions and gradually build up to 10 repetitions.

If you are able to perform Exercise 4 without difficulty (either or both of the alternatives) or after two or three weeks your hip pain is not decreasing when performing activities such as going up or down stairs or rising from a chair, progress on to Exercise 5.

Exercise 5: Hip strengthening in standing – two-legged half squat

Stand upright with your feet placed shoulder-width apart, a chair or stool behind you and an open door in front of you where you are able to grasp

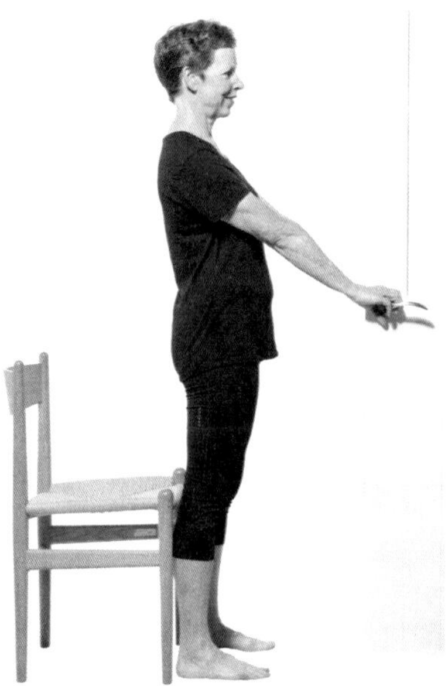

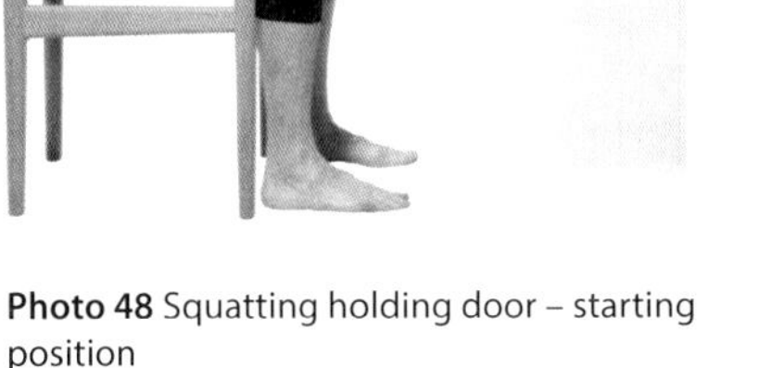

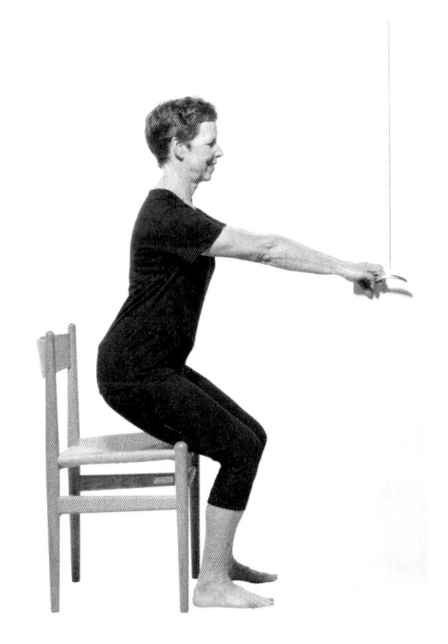

Photo 48 Squatting holding door – starting position

Photo 49 Squatting holding door

both door handles for support (*Photo 48*). Keep your feet flat on the floor, and slowly sit back towards the chair until you feel a firm tension in the muscles around your hips (*Photo 49*). Start with a small range of motion and do not sit on the chair. Hold this position for a few seconds, then return to the starting position.

Each time you perform this movement cycle try to keep your knees pointing forward, and lower your hips further until your buttocks are almost touching the back of the chair until you are able to perform this amount of controlled hip flexion with no hip pain.

Exercise 5 should be repeated 10 times per session two times a day – once in the morning and once in the afternoon or evening. Each time you repeat the exercise you must move to the edge of the pain and then release the pressure by returning to the starting position.

Once you can perform this exercise without difficulty over a few days or weeks, progress the exercise by performing the half squats without holding onto the door handle (*Photos 50 and 51*).

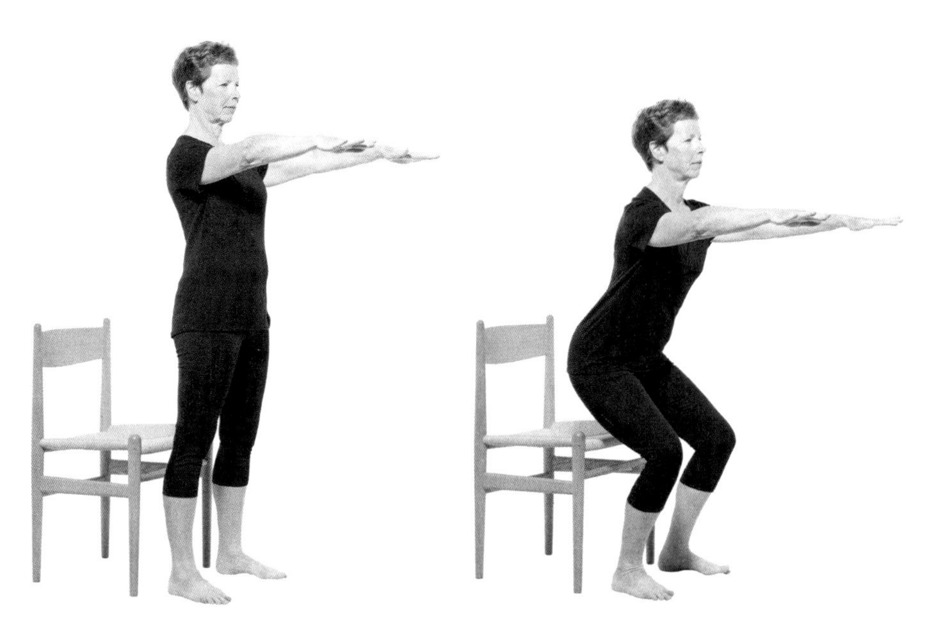

Photo 50 Squatting - starting position **Photo 51** Squatting

As your ability to perform this exercise improves, progress the number of repetitions until you are performing up to three sets of 15 repetitions twice a day.

By exercising this way you place the appropriate loading required to stimulate a recovery in the affected structures around your hip. Your pain should decrease over a few weeks as your hip regains its function-performing activities that requires your hip to take your body weight while bending.

Review your progress

We recommend in the case of lateral hip pain you perform Exercises 4 and 5 for up to six weeks to determine if the exercises are of benefit in reducing or abolishing your pain. A gradual decrease in pain when you perform activities such as going down hills, stairs, crouching or jumping indicates your hip pain is improving. In most cases the result eventually is a good recovery, however, progress can be slow, and it may be necessary to continue with Exercise 4 and Exercise 5 for up to three months as

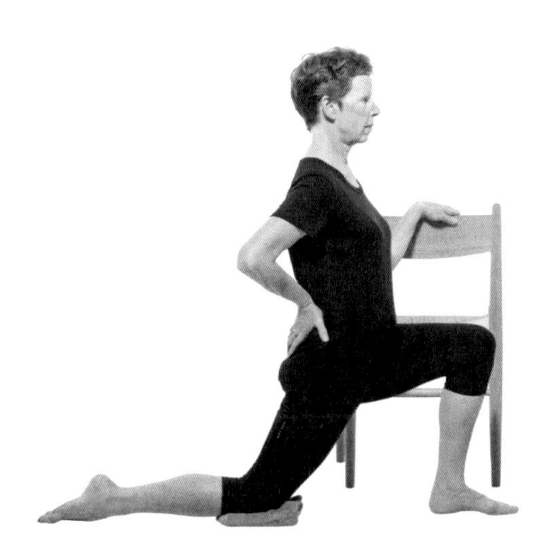

Photo 52 Hip extension in kneeling

some cases gradually improve over several months. Aim to reach the point where your affected hip and leg is as strong as your unaffected leg, and be prepared to resume the exercise programme if you feel your pain returning.

To prevent the recurrence of lateral hip pain, it is crucial to maintain your ability to perform exercises 4 and 5, and to continue good postures and positional habits for the hip as described in Chapter Three.

If you continue to have hip pain and a loss of function that is not resolving, we recommend that you contact a health-care professional who is fully qualified to provide the McKenzie Method®. These are members of the McKenzie Institute International who hold the Credentialing Certificate or the Diploma in Mechanical Diagnosis & Therapy®. To obtain the names of these treatment providers in your area we recommend that you use the search feature on the McKenzie Institute International website: www.mckenzieinstitute.org.

When you have no pain or stiffness

Many people with hip problems have lengthy spells in which they experience little or no pain. If you have ever had one or more episodes of hip pain you should start the exercise programme even though you may

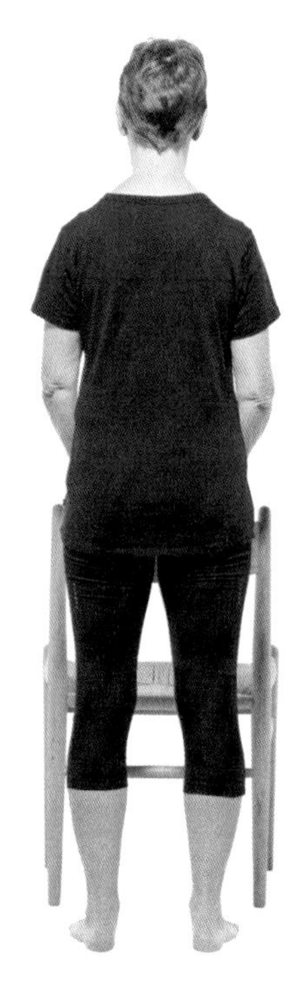

Photo 53 Hip abduction in standing

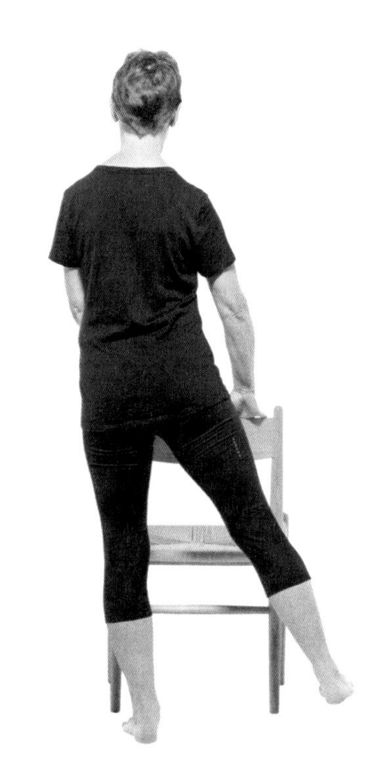

Photo 54 Hip abduction in standing

be pain-free at the moment. However, in this situation it is not necessary to do all the exercises or to exercise every two to three hours.

To prevent recurrence of hip problems you should perform Exercise 1: Hip extension in kneeling (*Photo 52*) two times a day to ensure you maintain your hip's range of motion.

If Exercise 4 or 5 has been the exercise sequence that has relieved your hip symptoms, perform these instead (*Photos 53 and 54 or 55 and 56*).

Furthermore, whenever you feel pain developing during activity or work you should perform these exercises. It is important you watch your hip postures at all times to ensure postural stresses are not the cause of hip pain. These exercises will have very little or no effect if you constantly fall back into your previous poor hip postures and prolonged static hip

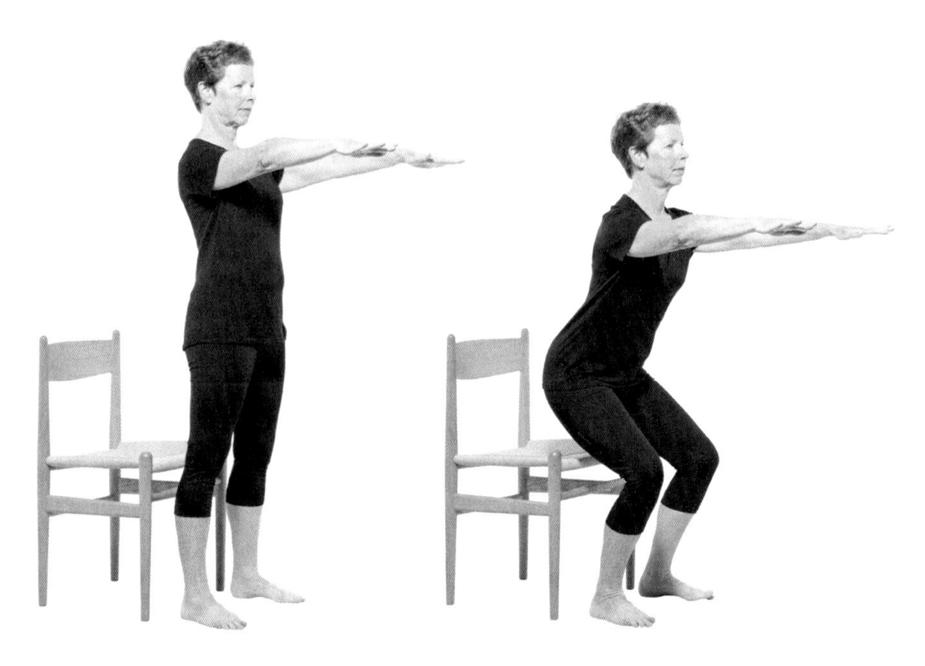

Photo 55 Two-legged half squat

Photo 56 Two-legged half squat

positions. While it may be advisable to exercise in the manner described above for the rest of your life, it is essential you develop and maintain good postural habits.

As it takes just a few minutes to perform one session of these exercises **don't let lack of time be an excuse for not doing these exercises**.

Yoga, pilates, tai chi and martial arts are activities that specifically promote postural awareness and provide exercises to ensure the hips and legs are put through a wide range of motion.

A graduated increase in activities that improves your fitness should also be considered. A regular walking, cycling or exercycle programme will assist in maintaining leg mobility; appropriately structured gym programmes and aerobics or fitness classes will assist with flexibility and strength at and around the hip. Further strategies to prevent recurrence are covered in Chapter Six.

Recurrence

At the first sign of recurrence of hip pain you should immediately perform the above exercises that have previously helped you.

If your pain is already too severe to tolerate these exercises or if they fail to reduce the pain, you must review the advice provided under acute management in Chapter Six, page 74. This will help you to determine when you can return to Exercise 1 and then gradually work through the exercise sequence again. Again, pay attention to your hip posture, regularly perform postural correction, and maintain the correct posture as much as you can when sitting, standing and lying.

Ongoing hip pain following hip surgery

Some people can experience ongoing hip pain or difficulty walking, rising from sitting or using stairs following hip replacement surgery or after suffering a fractured hip or pelvis. Walking in a swimming pool is an effective exercise to reduce pain and increase function as the water reduces the load through the hip by 50 per cent. **We recommend you obtain a medical clearance from your medical physician before commencing this programme.**

Commence with walking for five minutes, three days per week with one rest day between each, to establish a baseline of exercise that does not aggravate your hip pain. Gradually increase as comfort allows until you are able to walk 20–30 minutes at a time. It is usually necessary to continue this pool-walking programme for six weeks to experience lasting benefits. Exercises 4 and 5 can also be performed in the pool, but start cautiously, carefully following the instructions as above.

NOTES

Chapter 6: Acute management and prevention of recurrence

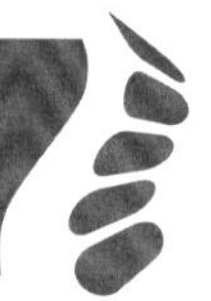

Acute management

If you have injured your hip within the past few days by twisting it or receiving a blow (in a fall, for example), it is possible you have injured the structures in and around the hip and triggered an inflammatory response, which is the body's response to injury. This inflammatory response can also be triggered by suddenly overstressing or overloading the hip without a specific injury or incident.

The hip will be painful at rest, and on moving it or attempting to take weight on that leg.

In the early stage it is necessary to reduce the effects of the injury by limiting any internal bleeding, swelling and pain through applying the regime: Protect, Optimal Loading, and Ice Therapy.

Protecting your hip from further damage is important for the first 24–48 hours by avoiding any activity that increases your pain and swelling. If you are limping when walking, the use of a walking stick will help to walk (short distances) more evenly and provide the optimal loading rather than being full weight-bearing (*Photo 57*). Use the stick in the opposite hand to the hip you have injured.

Apply a cold pack to your hip over the painful region for up to 15 minutes every three hours. To prevent an ice burn, place a damp towel or a thin layer of cooking or baby oil between your skin and the ice pack (*Photo 58*).

After 24 hours of applying treatment we recommend you cautiously commence the exercise programme in Chapter Five and follow the advice carefully. This will allow you to judge the optimal loading and also the correct direction of movement for your hip. Continue with the application of ice therapy for up to one week as required until the pain has reduced.

If it is too painful to perform the exercise programme, continue with Protect, Optimal Loading, and Ice Therapy regime for a further 24 hours then try again. If your hip is too painful to commence the exercise

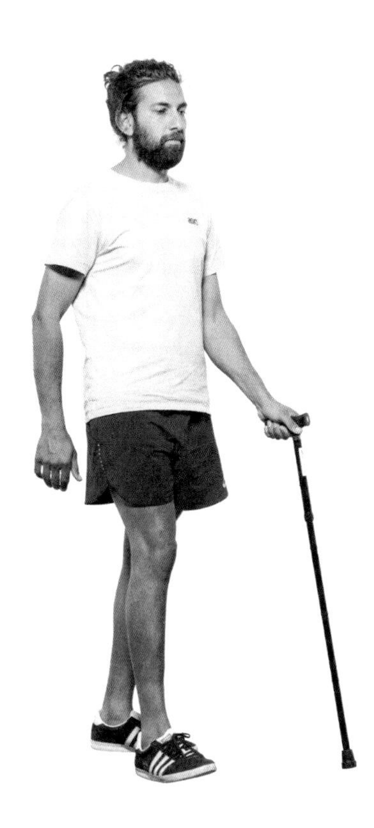

Photo 57 Walking with walking stick

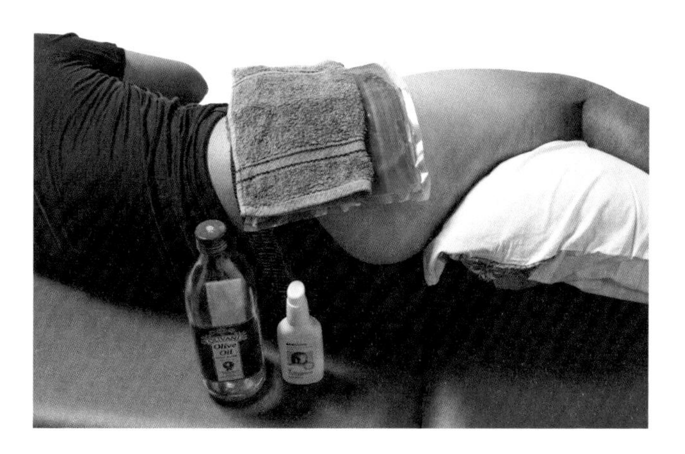

Photo 58 Apply an ice pack to your hip

programme after 48 hours we recommend you consult your doctor or physical therapist.

Prevention of recurrence

In earlier chapters we have discussed a specific exercise regime to follow to decrease pain, and increase flexibility and strength in your hip. However, we also discussed that exercises alone are only a part of the solution, and in order to **prevent** or **minimise** further episodes it is important to address the other aggravating factors that contribute to your hip pain.

The most important thing is to be more active, with walking, swimming or running, for example, and often losing some body weight. Cycling or use of an exercycle is another option for some people with hip pain, however ensure the seat is not too low as repeated hip flexion through the cycling motion can aggravate some hip conditions. But also bear in mind that if you already sit for long periods in other areas of your life, other recreational activities will get other parts of your body moving more.

This chapter aims to give you simple strategies to assist with changes of lifestyle that are an important part of breaking the cycle of recurrent hip pain. The strategies cover how to:

1. **interrupt prolonged sitting and standing postures regularly**
2. **increase the amount you walk**
3. **increase your general fitness**
4. **improve your balance**
5. **lose weight**

Most of these strategies are designed to be used in conjunction with the exercise programme described in this book to reduce the pain and improve the endurance, strength and function of your hip. Any movement or exercise is generally beneficial, provided you choose activities that do not make your hip pain worse, but, start cautiously. Some hip discomfort while exercising may be expected as long as it goes away afterwards. And if you do overexercise your hip and create more pain or swelling, refer back to the acute management section at the beginning of this chapter.

1. Interrupt prolonged sitting and standing postures regularly

Many of us have a sedentary job or lifestyle, and hours can pass before we realise we have not changed position, or we develop discomfort or pain that reminds us to move. This can also occur (less frequently) with prolonged standing.

The key is to move regularly before pain develops by building movement into your daily routines. There are several ways you can achieve this:

At work:

- ✓ Alternate between sitting and standing at an adjustable standing desk. Ask your employer if you are eligible for one, or consider buying one yourself.
- ✓ Use a printer that you have to walk to, rather than one directly by your desk.
- ✓ Set your software or cell phone to sound an alarm every 20 minutes or so to remind you to get up and stretch your legs with a short walk.
- ✓ Walk the long way to the cafe or lunch room during your work breaks.
- ✓ If it's difficult to get up, such as in a plane or car, try to stretch your legs out while sitting.
- ✓ If standing still and unable to walk around, march on the spot or do a few squats, holding on to a firm surface for support if necessary.

At home:

- ✓ Avoid a low chair. Ensure you sit in a firm chair at a height from which you can stand without too much effort – using your legs as much as possible, with minimal assistance from your arms if required.
- ✓ Leave the remote control at the opposite side of the room to your favourite seat so you have to get up and move when you want to use the remote control.

- ✓ If you are watching TV, get up and move about every time the advertisements come on.
- ✓ When on the phone, stand up rather than sit, perform your hip exercises or walk around.
- ✓ Set your software or cell phone to sound an alarm every 20 minutes or so to remind you to get up and stretch your legs with a short walk.
- ✓ Listen to music on vinyl rather than streaming. You have to get up every twenty minutes or so to turn the album over or change it.

2. Increase the amount you walk

Increasing your general level of walking is probably the single most important way of increasing your strength, endurance and balance in order to prevent or minimise recurrent hip pain. First, increase the number of minutes spent walking. These can be in one session, or accumulated over the day. Later you should increase the speed and even add some hills, being particularly cautious about adding in too much walking or hiking downhill, initially.

A good goal is 20–30 minutes of brisk walking 4–5 days per week. If your hip is painful or you are unfit, you may well need to start with less and let your body gradually adapt over several weeks. Do not increase your walking by more than 10 per cent from one session to the next. For example, if you have got used to 20 minutes of walking, progress to 22 minutes. Larger increases overstress the body and can aggravate your hip pain. What you don't want is to cause more pain that will put you off further exercise – otherwise you will return to the same cycle of losing fitness, putting on weight and continuing to have hip pain.

Ways to increase walking:

- ✓ Park your car at the far end of a carpark rather than taking the closest parking space to your destination. This is particularly true on a long car journey when you have pulled in for a break or coffee, etc.
- ✓ Get off the bus one stop earlier than usual and walk the rest of the way to your destination.
- ✓ Use the steps or stairs rather than the lift or escalator, for example, at a shopping mall or airport.

- ✓ Use your meal break at work for a walk, or walk the long way to your favourite or usual eating place.
- ✓ Begin a regular walking programme, preferably with a family member or friend to keep you motivated. Or join a local walking group.
- ✓ Buy or adopt a dog that you will have to take out for walks every day.
- ✓ Wear shoes that are comfortable and supportive. Try to walk on grass or tarmac rather than concrete, but be careful with uneven surfaces, which can be tough on your joints.
- ✓ Take a light to see and be seen if you are walking at night.
- ✓ Whilst walking, use the time listening to music or podcasts, learning a language, listening to a talking book, etc.
- ✓ Walking in a swimming pool is another good way to get started on a walking routine if your hips are painful initially. Walking in waist-deep water reduces load through the hip by 50 per cent.

3. Increase your general fitness

Once you are comfortable with a walking programme, you may feel confident to increase your general fitness by adding in other pursuits – either by gradually returning to previous recreational activities or taking up new interests. But start cautiously and slowly increase the intensity and the frequency. If you are over 55 years of age, or have underlying health conditions, we recommend that you consult with your own doctor or health-care professional about your exercise plans.

Ways to increase fitness:

- ✓ Start a graduated swimming or fitness routine, or join a local group or fitness club in your area.
- ✓ Get a bicycle, electric bike, mountain bike or exercycle and start a cycling routine. Or join a cycling club in your area.
- ✓ Resume activities that you have enjoyed in the past such as fitness classes, hiking, dancing or golf, for example.
- ✓ Take up an activity that you enjoy doing, have enjoyed in the past or have always thought about doing.
- ✓ Join a local gym and get a supervised graduated fitness programme.

Be cautious initially with any deep squatting or squats with weights if you are not used to it.

- ✓ Water-based activities such as pool walking or swimming are helpful if you have a limited walking capacity.

Injury prevention tips:

- ✓ We recommend you be able to walk comfortably for one hour before you consider higher impact activities such as jogging, tennis, or football that all involve some running. Running may be more risky for injury if you are overweight, and you will need to start cautiously, following these injury prevention tips even more carefully.
- ✓ Initially avoid running down hills as significantly increased loading is placed through your hips.
- ✓ Take time to warm up and cool down. The best way to warm up for an activity is to do the activity gently for the first five minutes. A cool down at the end, again doing the activity gently as you gradually slow down, keeps blood pumping back to the heart and vital organs as you recover.
- ✓ Give your body a chance to recover from exercise by taking days off. If you do high-impact activities, either rest or just do some easy walking or cycling to assist with the recovery the following day.
- ✓ Varying your activities has been shown to reduce overuse problems. Walk some days, swim or cycle other days. If weather or environmental factors are a problem, consider using equipment at home – a treadmill, an elliptical or cross-trainer machine or an exercycle. Often they can be borrowed or leased while you decide which is most suitable for you.
- ✓ Proper footwear is important, especially if walking or running on hard surfaces. And if possible run on grass in a park or a trail in the woods, rather than concrete as the loading stress through the hips is significantly less.

4. Improve your balance

There are simple ways to specifically stimulate the balance reactions in your hip joint – either when standing still or when on the move. Exercises 4 and 5 are effective in improving your balance as well as your strength,

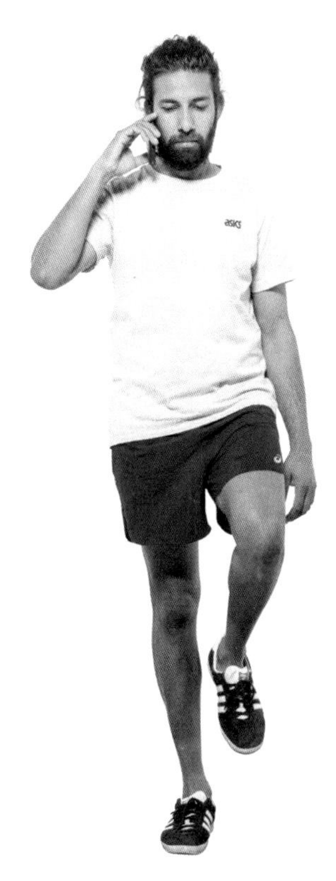

Photo 59 Balancing on one leg

and we give some other suggestions below. Further specific ways of improving your balance are tai chi classes run by community groups or health professionals.

Simple exercises:

- ✓ Balance on one leg when you brush your teeth, talk on the phone or stand doing a task at a bench, for example, cooking or washing the dishes etc. (*Photo 59*)
- ✓ Progress this by closing your eyes, rising onto your toes, or going into a slight squat on that leg.
- ✓ Sometimes go up or down stairs very slowly to challenge your strength and balance.

Before starting to use poles for walking and hiking consider whether you really need to use such walking aids. They are promoted as helping you feel more stable on uneven ground, or decreasing the load on the hip particularly walking downhill. But actually the opposite is required. It is better to improve your balance and hip function by gradually increasing the load on your hip with exercise, rather than over-protecting the hip and decreasing the load as a long-term solution. Once you start using a stick or pole you will become increasingly reliant on it.

5. Lose weight

Losing weight is achievable for most people. But, maintaining that weight loss is more difficult. Do NOT diet. Dieting is a short-term strategy, usually doomed to fail in the long term. Strive for a healthier lifestyle with moderate changes you can live with long term. To lose a significant amount of weight healthily takes 6–24 months. People who lose weight quickly tend to regain it with adverse effects on the metabolism. Aiming to lose a pound (half a kilo) a week on a consistent basis is a reasonable and obtainable goal. Portion control has been shown to be more effective when combined with exercise.

We recommend you seek advice from your doctor or attend a recognised weight-loss programme should you have underlying health issues or seek to lose a significant amount of weight.

Top tips to lose weight:

- ✓ Eat less each meal (smaller portions) – even if you do not immediately change the food you are eating. Reduce the size of your meals by 25 per cent, or stop eating when you are 75 per cent full. Within 20 minutes the food will expand in your body and you will feel satisfied.
- ✓ Researchers have found overweight people eat more quickly. Slow down and give the food a chance to register and expand in your stomach.
- ✓ Stop eating unhealthy snacks, for example chocolate, sweet snacks, crisps.
- ✓ Eat a more balanced diet including a greater percentage of fruit and vegetables.
- ✓ Drink more water, but less alcohol, soda pops/fizzy drinks, which have a high sugar content.

- ✓ Order less food in restaurants. Split a meal with a friend, order fewer courses, or ask for a container for you to take away any excess food when you have had sufficient.
- ✓ Do not shop when hungry. You will make poor choices. Avoid having unhealthy food in the house.

The key thing to consider is that changes to your lifestyle and general fitness need to be gradually implemented in order to be sustainable. However, by following the instructions and information in this book you have every opportunity to participate in an active, healthy lifestyle in order to remain pain free, or minimise further episodes of hip pain.

Should you require, or would prefer, to have a McKenzie assessment before commencing any of the exercises described in Chapter Five or the fitness strategies discussed in this chapter, we recommend that you contact a health-care professional who is fully qualified to provide the McKenzie Method. These are members of the McKenzie Institute International who hold the Credentialing Certificate or the Diploma in Mechanical Diagnosis & Therapy®. To obtain the names of these treatment providers in your area we recommend that you use the search feature on the McKenzie Institute International website: www.mckenzieinstitute.org.

NOTES

References

Alentorn-Geli E, Samuelsson K, Musahl V, et al. (2017)
'The Association of Recreational and Competitive Running With Hip and Knee Osteoarthritis: A Systematic Review and Meta-analysis'. *Journal of Orthopeadic and Sports Physical Therapy*, 47, 6, pp.373–390.

Bennell K, Hinman R (2011)
'A review of the clinical evidence for exercise in osteoarthritis of the hip and knee'. *Journal of Science and Medicine in Sport*, 14, pp.4–9.

Cibulka M, Bloom N, Enseki K, et al.(2017)
Hip Pain and Mobility Deficits—Hip Osteoarthritis: Clinical Practice Guidelines Linked to the International Classification of Functioning, Disability and Health From the Orthopaedic Section of the American Physical Therapy Association. *Journal of Orthopeadic and Sports Physical Therapy*, 47, 6, pp.A1–A37.

Fransen M, McConnell S, Hernandez-Molina G, Reichenbach S (2014)
'Exercise for osteoarthritis of the hip'. *Cochrane Database Systematic Reviews*, 4, Article No. CD007912.

Silvis M, Mosher T, Smetana B, et al. (2011)
'High Prevalence of Pelvic and Hip Magnetic Resonance Imaging Findings in Asymptomatic Collegiate and Professional Hockey Players'. *American Journal of Sports Medicine*, 39, 4, pp.715–721.

Svege I, Nordsletten L, Fernandes L, Risberg MA (2015)
'Exercise Therapy May Postpone Total Hip Replacement Surgery in Patients with Hip Osteoarthritis: a Long-Term Follow-Up of a Randomised Trial'. *Annals of the Rheumatic Diseases*, 74,1, pp.164–9.

Zhang W, Moskowitz RW, Nuki G, et al. (2008)
'Oarsi Recommendations for the Management of Hip and Knee Osteoarthritis, Part II: Oarsi Evidence-Based, Expert Consensus Guidelines'. *Osteoarthritis Cartilage*, Feb, 16, 2, pp.137–62.

https://www.telegraph.co.uk/news/health/news/7738663/Britons-spend-more-than-14-hours-a-day-sitting-down.html

https://www.dailymail.co.uk/health/article-2321784/Two-thirds-Britons-spend-20-HOURS-day-sitting-lying-down.html

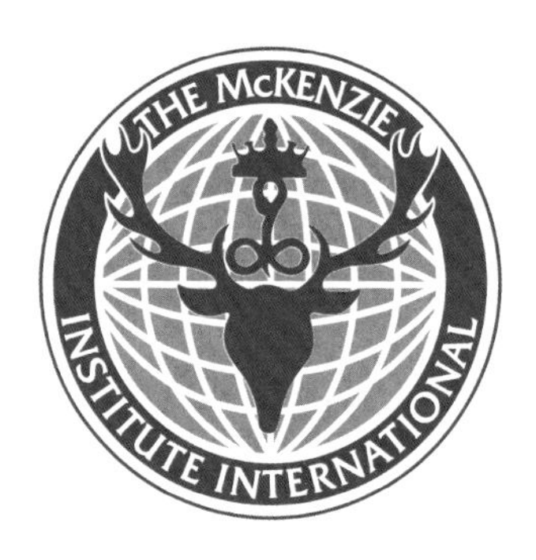

The McKenzie Institute International®

The McKenzie Institute International Head Office website:

www.mckenzieinstitute.org

Includes information about:

- Robin McKenzie
- The McKenzie Method of Mechanical Diagnosis and Therapy®
- The McKenzie Institute International
- The McKenzie Institute's Education Programme

Can help you find:

- Certified McKenzie Clinics
- Diplomaed and Credentialled McKenzie therapists
- Your local branch

The McKenzie Institute International Head Office

3 Alexander Road, PO Box 2026,
Raumati Beach 5255, New Zealand

Website: **www.mckenzieinstitute.org**
Email: **headoffice@mckenzieinstitute.org**
Phone: **+64 4 299-6645** Facsimile: **+64 4 299-7010**

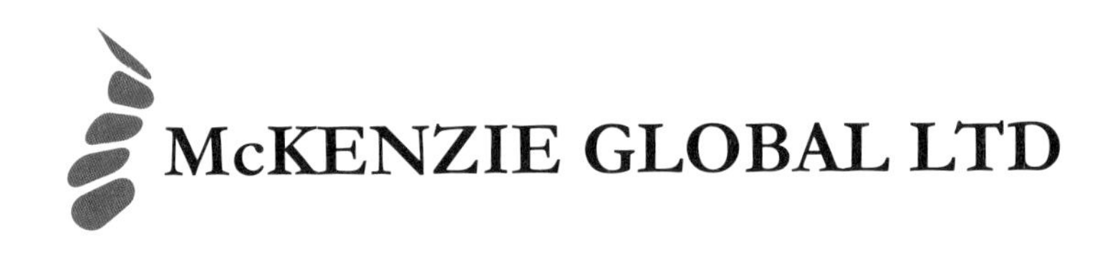

Robin McKenzie's patient handbooks, Treat Your Own Back, Treat Your Own Neck, Treat Your Own Shoulder, Treat Your Own Knee and Treat Your Own Hip, along with The Original McKenzie® lumbar and cervical supports are available in the U.S. and Canada from OPTP.com.

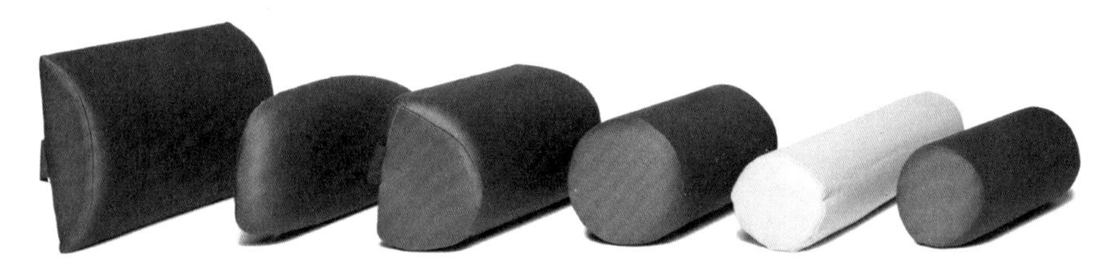

The Original McKenzie® Products

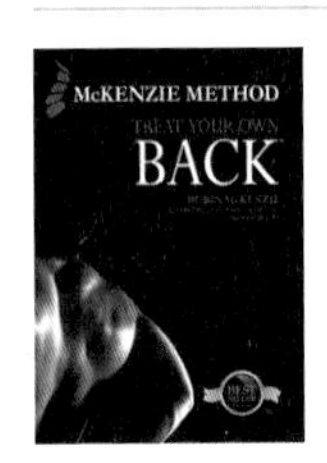

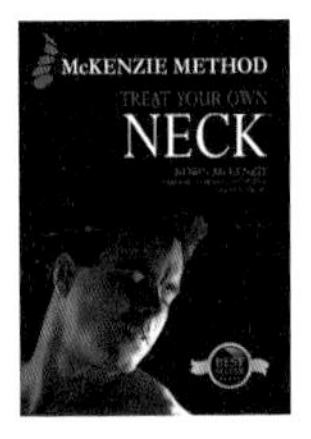

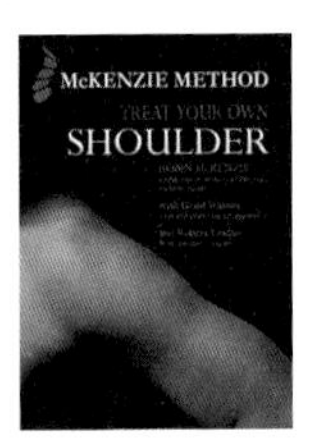

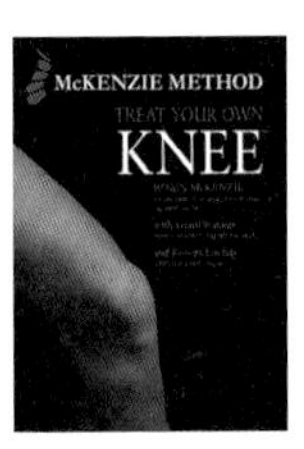

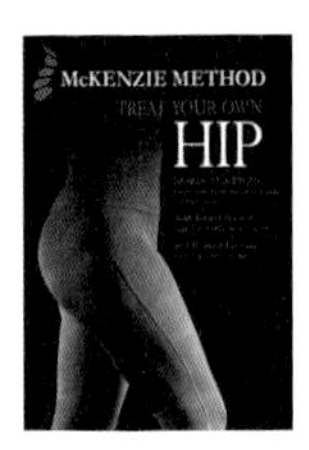

E-Book editions now available.

Exclusively distributed by OPTP in the U.S. and Canada.

Order at **OPTP.com** or call **800-367-7393**

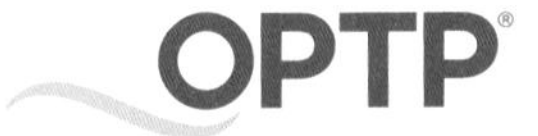

TOOLS FOR FITNESS. KNOWLEDGE FOR HEALTH.